CURE YOURSELF
NATURALLY

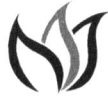

CURE YOURSELF NATURALLY

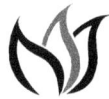

WHAT TO DO WHEN YOUR DOCTOR CANNOT HEAL YOU

BY GINA KOPERA, M.H.

COUNCIL BLUFFS, IOWA

WARNING: None of the statements in this book have been evaluated or approved by the Food and Drug Administration or the American Medical Association. The information provided is intended for your general knowledge only and is not a substitute for professional medical advice or treatment for specific medical conditions. Always seek the advice of your physician or other qualified health care provider before using any herbal products.

Manufactured in the United States of America

For inquiries contact:

Gina Kopera
2704 2nd Avenue
Council Bluffs, IA 51501
gina@ginascorner.com
www.ginascorner.com

Book edited & designed by Erin Zimmer www.designer-editor.com

Cover Design by Brian J. Craft grandanvil@cox.net

ISBN-10: 1-44-863779-1
ISBN-13: 978-1-448-63779-9

DEDICATED TO MY FATHER

Table of Contents

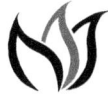

Acknowledgments

I am pleased to have the privilege of writing this page, and I am so grateful for everyone that was in my life through this process of putting this book together. Thank you for your patience. I am sure many can recite this entire book, and the words, "It is finally over!" are music in your ears. Yeah!

First and foremost I acknowledge my father and mother. Thank you for creating me. I love you both. Thank you for believing in me. After all, this is entirely my father's fault; he was the one that planted the seed. It simply took me awhile to water it.

This would not have been possible if it was not for the support of my husband and son. They lived through all my many fasts and cleansings, and they even put up with me talking about poop all hours of the day and night.

I am grateful to my very first editor, Jan Lund, for her patience with me through the years of starting and stopping my story.

This would of never of happened if it were not for my teachers. There are not enough words to express my appreciation for their educational support and influence in helping me learn about the natural healing of the body and mind. Thank you, Dr. Christopher, Dr. Schulze, Dr. Hulda Clarke, Dr. Crook, Sam Biser, Dr. James Balch, Phyllis Balch, F. Batmanghelidj M.D., Wayne Dyer, Dr. Welbe, Dr. Lorraine Day, Joyce Meyer and The School of Natural Healing, and David and Fawn Christopher.

and

All of my clients, they are great teachers for me to teach others…

Of course, then there are my friends and family, which I kept at the phone for unlimited hours. This is where the encouragement to keep my head up and courage to get this all put together came from. Sheila Luhr-Kuhn, Rita Griffin, Carla Lyons, Julie Marella, Tammy Brackett, Shariee McClendon and my family.

I am eternally grateful to Erin Zimmer for being the brilliant editor of this book, for her expertise in editing, design, and guidance. You can reach her at www.designer-editor.com.

Forward From Dad

It was in April of 2000 when Gina came to our house in Arizona from her home in Iowa with her young son, Devin. She was obviously extremely distraught, and her world was crashing down. It was then that we had a "dad-daughter talk" like when she was a little girl. She relayed to me that, among other problems, she had MS. She was taking $800 of drugs a month – four shots at $200 each. Her left side was numb, she had a hard time opening a car door, and her sight was going bad, amongst other symptoms.

This conversation terrified me since my mother had MS. She was an invalid for many years and died a horrible death as a result of treatments for MS and cancer, which she contracted in the later years of her life. I certainly hoped my daughter would not take the same path.

The next couple of days, we talked about what could be accomplished by changing eating habits and reducing stress. I introduced her to Vicki, who had an office next to ours. Vicki was told she had three months to get her life in order because she would soon be wheelchair-bound. Instead of succumbing to MS, she researched the disease and then changed her diet. She found that gluten was the main culprit and eliminated from her diet. Today, she is more robust than ever before.

I also introduced Gina to Greta, a very good friend and an expert in the health field. She too, stated that gluten was to be avoided and encouraged the 'no drug' approach to good health.

I encouraged Gina to conquer MS, rather than live with it: I suggested for her to research two prominent experts in the field of Natural Healing and I gave her Sam Biser's books and videos, and suggested she go to his website at www.sambiser. com. I also asked her to go to Dr. Lorraine Day's website at www.drday.com.

Gina not only went to these websites and read the Sam Biser book I gave her, she went much further. Gina is living proof that MS can be licked. Further, she is now my guiding light to healthier living. I am extremely proud of her.

I am also very grateful for the support from the people around her. I am especially grateful to Greg, her husband, and Devin, her son and my grandson. The support of family and friends is extremely important to recovery.

Gina has exceeded my expectations. She is an inspiration to anyone who prefers health over sickness.

INTRODUCTION

This book is about my desire to seriously inspire you to journey into natural healing. I did not go searching for this experience. It was thrust upon me after traveling through a nightmarish experience of debilitating illness and personal conflict, from which I now have the expertise to guide you and to help remove the confusion surrounding natural healing.

At one point I was on the verge of being penniless, driven there by being insurance poor, medical poor, and even health-food store poor. My determined effort to cure my long and involved illnesses drained every dollar I had.

But where I once suffered, there is now deep knowledge. I know all the sacrifice was worth it because I can now help you save money and even save your life. You don't have to be educated or rich. This road to health is accessible for everyone!

I know, through the many people I come in contact with, that we are floundering to understand symptoms and diseases with names that we cannot pronounce clearly and have to look up their definitions.

I am here to take the confusion out of natural healing. You don't have to get lost anymore, as my approach is very easy. This is where getting healthy becomes simple again. The same three steps are the foundation used for healing any disease: Cleanse, Nourish and Let Thy Body Heal Itself. I will even show you how to make your own products, if you choose.

> **Chapters 1 through 5** are about my personal journey. I like to think I am perfect…but I am not. At times when I was going through my agonizing nightmares, I did not take control of my health, nor did I even care. I believe this is critical for you to know and understand.
>
> I was given a huge compliment by several people years ago after developing the PowerHouse fast and cleansing. "Wow, Gina must have really healed herself with that fast. The way she has been taking care of herself and not even getting sick is remarkable," they said.
>
> A few years after that grand cleanse, again going through a very difficult time in my personal life, caused me to "fall off the wagon." Into what, you ask?
>
> Simple: indulging in old comfort habits.

Even so, my health had become so good that my body didn't have another symptom. This is how powerful the "cleanse and nourish" healing has worked, even years later. It will strengthen and tone your weak areas, especially in your time of need.

These statements about me apply to a great many people, people just like YOU.

Chapters 6 through 11 are full of information you need about your body and nutrition. There are things that are good for your body and things that are bad for it. Understand how your body works and you will be half way towards healing. These chapters cover everything from organ functions to Candida infections to parasites. And more!

Chapters 12 through 20 detail everything you need to know to successfully complete cleansing your body of toxins and fasting for nourishment and recovery. Would you get a new car and never change the oil? I think not! Just like maintaining your car, your organs need to be flushed out. Get excited for yourself for this incredible journey you are about to embark on. It is exciting, all the changes your body is going to go through and how much power you have now under your own fingertips. These protocols will help you, from your hooter to your tooter, get back to health.

The good news is: we can all get back into the saddle and continue with positive health, taking full advantage of remarkable opportunities that are right at our fingertips. Thank you for reading my book. I know the journey you are about to take will change your life for the better – forever.

MY STORY OF REGAINING HEALTH FOR MY SON AND MYSELF

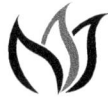

CHAPTER 1

THE ONSET OF MS

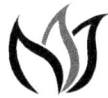

At 21, having graduated from cosmetology school and with the intent of striking out on my own, I moved to Omaha, Nebraska, leaving behind the sunny climes of Phoenix. In those first three years, I met and fell in love with my husband. We were married five months after we met.

After marriage began on another new phase of life: starting my own nail salon and gift shop. My husband, a successful construction business owner, helped me by building-out my new shop just the way I envisioned. Together, we created a warm, inviting, and efficient atmosphere for my business to take hold. And take hold it did!

At 24, I was off and running with a future as bright as any star in the night sky. My clientele and inventory grew exponentially. Happy, fulfilled, successful, and three short years later, pregnant! Our plans included building our own little dream house. Things were shaping up like clockwork: I was the thrilled mom of a sweet, beautiful baby boy.

Like many other women, I was busy juggling the various roles of wife, new mother, and successful business entrepreneur. At 27, I was a manicurist/nail tech with a full Rolodex of my own clients, but also the "boss" in charge of hiring and firing, the buyer of the gift inventory, the display and design specialist, and the gift-shop sales person. From keeping the books to buying advertising, and I oversaw to the day-to-day running of my own Nail Gallery Empire! But this happy reality was very much in jeopardy.

I started to experience symptoms common to MS, including dizziness, weakness, numbness in the limbs, a sensation of tingling pins and needles, and blurred vision. After a series of diagnostic test procedures, I was diagnosed with the disease in June 1997. The doctor told me I would go home and cry my eyes out; I left feeling hopeless. My condition was labeled as "remitting and relapsing." The intermittent nature of my symptoms allowed me to go into a period of denial, ignoring the whole thing for almost a year.

When the symptoms returned a year later, I sought a second opinion, just to make sure the diagnosis was correct. I was referred to the top hospital in the area UMC (University Medical Center) which has a department called The MS Center. I thought they would be more understanding, which was important to me since I wasn't very comfortable with the previous neurologist I went to. He came up with the same diagnosis of MS but didn't want to put me in the actual category of "remitting and relapsing" quite yet, deciding to wait until I had more symptoms... which happened six months later. See Appendix B for my actual medical records documenting my condition at the time.

During this period, seeking for solace and support of others with MS, I joined a support group locally and online, surfed the Web for insight and sympathy, walked in the Race For The Cure in Chicago (where I raised an awesome amount of money, if I do say so myself), and generally made myself aware of the current medical procedures and prognoses available.

As I educated myself about the disease, I constantly ran up against an aura of pessimism. The prevailing attitude was, while MS was not a death sentence, per-se, it inevitably leads to a life of incapacity in a wheelchair or worse. People everywhere with MS were planning their existence around the fact they had a disease that would rob them of their vitality, their control, and their dignity. Clearly they felt I should start preparing for that day, myself. How life would or should be lead from a wheelchair was predominant, even before that 'inevitability' had come.

It's not that I didn't think about it. Sure, numbness and weakness, especially in my hands, the use of which my professional life depended upon, loomed as bad news for me. But preparation for being wheelchair-bound was not on my radar screen, not yet at least. Or was it? I was alarmed to discover that was exactly what I had begun to do! I imagined my husband needing to run my business, along with his own, to care for our child all by himself and, worse yet, to care for me.

This was an unbearable vision, so I made the decision to close my wonderful shop. There was some space in a beauty shop around the corner where I could still work but cut my hours back. I rested and planned out my remaining time of relatively good health, uncertain if it would be years, months, or mere weeks.

In the Throes of MS

My symptoms intensified. Finally my doctor put me on Avonex, one of the drugs in the interferon-beta family. When I first started this drug I felt as if I was having a heart attack! Two months later, I was in misery. Optic neuritis developed in my left eye. I also had extensive tingling and numbness, which are typical MS symptoms.

I was given 5000 mg. of corticosteroids in five days, the theory being that the tingling and numbness were due to inflammation in my neck. The steroids did not prove effective and, in the meantime, the Avonex treatment was as debilitating to me as chemotherapy often is to cancer sufferers. I was beginning to question whether the cure was worse than the disease!

For one to two days after each weekly shot of Avonex, I was incapacitated, needing to sleep most of the time in order to recuperate. And, because a typical side effect of interferon meds is severe depression, I had to go on anti-depressants, as well. Talk about depression: my insurance went up $600 the first two years, and $800 subsequently for each of the next four years.

I was on Avonex for fourteen months and I felt my whole world was revolving around MS. The prophecy had indeed become self-fulfilling. I was figuratively and literally in a dizzying descent — an ever-increasing downward spiral.

My work situation, almost exactly mimicking my health situation, was taking a major turn for the worse, too. My future career outlook loomed as bleakly as the past had been bright. Closing my shop and moving in with the hair salon had been a huge mistake—one that could not be undone. I internalized all of my worry, hurt, and pain about work and my ever-widening panorama of MS symptoms, and I comforted myself each night…with food.

Down and Out in the Land of MS

I cannot put my finger with certainty on any one cause of what happened next, but it doesn't take the proverbial Ph.D. to figure it out: my home life began to crash in around me. Whether due to or in spite of MS, I began to go through the most horrific stress of my life. This manifested itself in my sleeping, at most, one to two hours per night, for almost two months. Without realizing it, I had nearly stopped eating. I went – accidentally! – On what could only be described as an unintentional cleansing fast. I didn't know that I was fasting, didn't even know what fasting was. I just knew I couldn't even think about eating.

Things at home had gotten so bad that I temporarily walked away from my business, from my husband, and left town, taking our little boy with me. I had to get away. I needed my family and a safe place to think and recover, so I went back home to Arizona for two weeks.

Remarkably, in the midst of all this upheaval, my symptoms disappeared. Although stress is said to exacerbate MS, this unbelievably horrific stress had seemingly wiped it out. The MS symptoms went away along with other things that I knew weren't right, such as bumps (they looked like pimples) on the backs of my upper arms; I had experienced those since childhood, and now they were gone. Until that time, I had always felt thick and bloated. Food didn't process well after I ate. After the fast, I was no longer bloated, food went through my system easily, and the constant desire to eat was gone. I began to get my domestic life back in order, for which I am very thankful: I stopped taking drugs and steroids, and seemed to be on the rebound to good health.

The Road Back

At the time of my "accidental fast," I began to have inkling about the role food played in my cycle of symptoms. When I was eating breakfast again, the tingling would reappear by noon, so I stopped eating that meal. In addition, I added exercise and did not consume any alcohol. I stayed symptom-free! It was August of 2000 and I was doing yoga, other exercises, maintaining my low weight (I had dropped five dress sizes) and feeling good.

Things were back to normal; I was in Omaha again with my husband and child. Our marriage was much improved and we decided to take a well-deserved second honeymoon in Cancun, Mexico. In vacation mode, I ate more in one week than I had in months and had the occasional alcoholic drink too. When we returned from that trip, I began to experience dizzy spells and vertigo severe enough to bring on nausea. The logical conclusion seemed I had an intolerance to alcohol, which caused my MS symptoms to flare. I excluded it from my diet without a problem.

I decided to try to "cleanse" and "detox" my body with a one-day fast, in February 2001. All of the symptoms I had at that time promptly went away and stayed away. It was about at this time I began to hear of diets that were wheat and gluten free. I decided to take myself off of wheat, to see how I would like it. However, because I still ate oatmeal daily, a source of protein similar to gluten, the "experiment" failed.

By May 2001, I was experiencing weakness. In June, another seemingly innocuous decision turned out to be a crux for beginning to use some naturalistic healing practices. I had an IUD inserted. Call it fate, synchronicity, or serendipity, the day I got the IUD put in I happened to also have a cold sore on my lip and my father was in town. How did these events tie together?

A year or more prior to my worst moments of despair, my father had sent me the book *Saving Your Life with Cayenne* by Sam Biser. This book is an interview with Dr. Schulze, a Master Herbalist. It is filled with his experiences and teaches others how to go about healing themselves. Dr. Schulze was a student of the late Dr. Christopher, who I will tell you more about later.

Now, I love my Dad, but he had been on these "tangents" before. (Remember the nutritionists-instead-of-back-surgery incident?) I respected him, but I didn't always give his ideas the attention I now know they merited.

To be honest, when I opened the box and saw a book that said *Saving Your Life with Cayenne*, I rolled my eyes, thought "Okaaaayyyy," put it away, and didn't think about it again until about a year later. My mind was not closed to the idea of holistic or natural medicine, but to fight this disease, I trusted what I knew at the time: conventional medicine. I never had read the book Dad sent, but found the bottle of cayenne tincture he had left when visiting. He had learned how to make the cayenne tincture from Sam Biser's book. My father gave me the low-down on what it did, and then added, "When something is ill, it has a lack of circulation, so cayenne it."

I was not familiar with cayenne, but I did know that the $50 cold-sore ointment and the dollar-a-day pills I had been prescribed weren't working. I decided to try the tincture of cayenne that my Dad had offered. Overnight, the cold sore was scabbed and healed. It never even festered. I was impressed but I still was not seeing the big picture.

The IUD started giving me problems, which in turn triggered MS symptoms. A low-grade infection was diagnosed and persisted. Finally, I had the IUD removed less than a month after its insertion. That doctor told me MS symptoms could not be connected with the IUD. But, contrary to what he thought, the truth is that any infection in the body can exacerbate the symptoms of MS.

After the IUD was removed, scar tissue remained, undetected by blood tests, urine tests, or ultrasound. I was weak, bleeding frequently, and spending a lot of time lying on the couch. This gave me the time and impetus to read, and I started with Sam Biser's book on the healing properties of cayenne.

In his book, I read a case study about a woman who had uterine cancer that was causing a lot of bleeding. When she douched with cayenne tincture, her bleeding stopped immediately. At that time I was getting so sick — and desperate — I decided to try what was described in that chapter of Biser's book. I went home, made up a formula according to the measurements given, and administered it to myself.

The moment I did that was the moment the bleeding stopped! This is when my skepticism began to abate and I sat down to seriously read Sam Biser's book. I went to Great Plains Labs and had a complete battery of tests run for wheat, gluten, and lactose intolerance. I eliminated grains and dairy from my diet definitively. Things were going well until I experienced another bout of optic neuritis. This time, since I was becoming more cognizant of the food link to symptom alleviation, I went to the health food store seeking something that might help my eyes. Lutein was suggested and I started having positive results the very day I began taking it.

The first day I could see the green glow coming from my alarm clock: this became my vision test every morning! The next day, when I woke up, I checked my left eye and found that I could make out one number. The following day, I could see two numbers, and so it went. Every single day, I reached some new landmark in my recovery, and by the time I had been on Lutein for two weeks, my eye problems had cleared up.

Even after my eyesight returned, however, July of 2001 found me battling again with MS symptoms. This time, my left hand was completely devoid of feeling and control of the fingers. Upset and dejected, I put in a call to the MS specialist. It was a Friday night, so I had to speak with someone on call. No one returned my phone call, so on Saturday I waited until noon, figuring they were busy. I finally got a hold of someone who said that, even though this seemed like an emergency to me, the emergency room personnel would not consider it one and that I would need to have an MS doctor consult. But he did suggest that their 24-hour lab could run the necessary blood and urine tests for infection, and those results would speed things up, come Monday, when I could see my doctor. I agreed and went in for those tests.

Early Monday morning, I took my son to the daycare and cleared my calendar, since I reasoned that I would need to be ready to go in first thing and get back on the steroid treatment. I wasn't looking forward to going back on that treatment, but if it was the only thing a person in my situation could do, I was willing to do anything! After all, my profession depended on my being able to control my fingers; at that moment, I couldn't even make a fist.

All that Monday morning, I waited for a call. Hour after hour ticked by but, even though I left messages, no one returned my call. By noon, I was sitting in my house and crying when it suddenly dawned on me: I was the only one sitting around crying over my condition. No one else was paying the slightest attention to my problem.

I dried my tears and said to myself, "Gina, figure it out. Think! Find out what you can do for yourself." That's when I took charge of my own treatments. This time, I was on a quest. I did deeper and more serious research, determined to come to some reliable conclusions. I had already read about fasting, so I decided to start with that. I went to the grocery store and got everything Phyllis A. Balch called for in her book Prescription for Nutritional Healing.

Around four in the afternoon, the doctor's office did finally call me back, and made an appointment for me for the following Friday. By that point I had decided on a complete detoxification of my entire body. To that end, I started the fasting protocols outlined in Ten-day Live Juice Fast by Balch & Balch, which is a basic prescription for nutritional healing. By this juncture, I was already 80% vegetarian, and wheat and gluten-free. Within 15 hours on the live juice fast I could make a fist with my left hand! This was great news because it meant that I would be able to go back to work. I was on the way to finding my way back to a healthy body and happy life.

When my Friday doctor's appointment finally arrived I had regained the total use of my hand. The doctor was very surprised at this, and ordered an MRI. I canceled that appointment at the end of the ten-day fast; I was completely symptom-free except for some slight numbness in a couple of fingertips.

In January 2002, I felt the onset of eye discomfort after a month of eating a few too many holiday sweets, so I did another ten-day fast. Within the first day of the fast, the discomfort in my eye was gone, but I decided to continue with the full ten days because fasts were supposedly beneficial in prevention too. Again, I was left with just a slight numbness in two fingers.

In March of 2002, I had been nearly symptom free, the exception being the numbness in those two fingertips, which I looked on as a gentle reminder. The major symptoms had been gone long enough for me to believe the steps I had taken, the diet I had followed, and the books I had read could benefit other MS sufferers. I was invited to share my experiences at a local MS support group. Within a day or two of my presentation, I received a letter in the mail from the facilitators who felt obligated to somehow "clear up [my] thinking about alternative medicine." In other words, telling me to stop promoting the benefits of herbal and natural remedies, diet, and detoxification to people who needed medication.

After the facilitators had their say, I was left with a feeling of sadness for them. True to form, they were in the business of promoting a "life" that revolved around the illness. I began to have distinct regrets about ever having been sucked into that negative thinking. It was not supportive. It promoted a pessimistic view of no hope and no "out." But it was true that I had, sadly, bought into that at one time. After being diagnosed with MS I had given up the hope of having more children. Now, knowing that I could live a life relatively free of the disease, I regretted terribly that I had abandoned my life's dream of having a slew of kids.

But no more regrets! The journey of a lifetime had begun — with the proverbial single step. And the one thing I had learned from the whole experience was precisely what positive people always say: Hang on tight to your dreams and do what you want to do. I wanted to live for today, not yesterday or tomorrow. And I was on my way to doing just that.

First Conclusion

I discovered a clear link between a healthy diet and MS symptom abatement. As things stand for me today, because of a series of events (sometimes horrific) that led me to fasting and detoxifying my body, I am as healthy as I've been in years.

Starting thousands of years ago, and continuing throughout many cultures around the world today, people have believed that we can close the gap between humans and the natural world in order to live better, healthier lives. Many theories exist (macrobiotics, for one) which suggest that sickness and unhappiness are nature's way of urging us to adopt a proper diet and way of life. These are not related to "new age" or fad diet philosophies; they are very much mainstream. Decades ago two publications, Dietary Goals for the United States (1977) and Diet, Nutrition and Cancer (1982) endorsed sweeping dietary changes for this country.

Sam Biser's book, Saving Your Life with Cayenne, was the greatest influence in my life. I can't imagine where I would be today without that information. Through its advice I have learned to treat many ailments besides just cold sores, such as: headaches, fatigue, bladder infection, cold and flu symptoms, etc.

CHAPTER 2

BETTER BUT NOT THERE YET

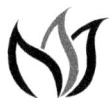

I knew what a fast was, I knew how to juice, and I knew that my symptoms of MS were abating. I had been teeter tottering back and forth with the fasting. The very first fast I had done was the recipe out of Prescriptions for Nutritional Healing. It was a fast that consisted of the live juice of raw vegetables (which I jokingly referred to as swamp water), and it tasted just awful. But I received tremendous benefits from it!

This led me to doing more reading and finding out about the different types of fasting recipes. I added in grape or apple juice. This greatly improved the taste, but I was not receiving the healing I expected. I received some health improvements, true, but still had some numbness in my hands. More importantly, even with everything I tried, I would eventually become ill again and have to look for a new fast.

I did a whole series of lemonade fasts next, with lemon, maple syrup and cayenne. That tasted a lot better! This fasting, like the previous ones, would work for a bit, but it would never pull me far enough. Then I found the watermelon fast. I juiced it and discovered that watermelon is a great diuretic and also a nutritious food. But the fasts of juice that tasted good weren't working on a permanent basis. I had to find something else.

I turned next to carrots and apples, thinking I would be getting more nutrition. I went on a twenty-four-day fast of this, and all I lost was eight pounds, which didn't seem right. I felt I had about twenty to twenty-five pounds of excess weight on me, and I had expected it to drop right off, but it didn't. I eventually even began to get MS symptoms again. My sight would go or more numbness would come. I would immediately stop what I was doing and start a new fast but the health improvements would only last for a few months.

Fasting Was Not Enough

At that point in time, I had also been vegetarian for two years, and I drank plenty of water, the uncontrollable weight gain just didn't make any sense to me. I kept thinking, "Does this fasting have something to do with my metabolism? Could I have messed it up by fasting?" I couldn't control the weight. And then, one day, someone suggested that I add some meat back into my diet. They told me it would help me to lose the excess weight.

I had been eating no meat for years, so when I did add it back in, it was in the form of a little bit of chicken in a salad. The very next day, I dropped seven pounds! My energy level also began coming up. I had been getting really tired by two or three o'clock, every day, but with the addition of meat back into my diet, that fatigue vanished.

My husband had a good analogy for this: Humans, like other meat-eating animals in the animal kingdom, have eyeteeth in addition to their flat molars. Animals that eat grass have flat teeth. If we have pointed teeth, it must be that we are designed to eat meat. It made sense! That is what led me to Sally Fallon's book, Nourishing Traditions.

I did not give up fasting, but I now understood that meat was meant to be part of my life. About this time, I also discovered raw milk. I had read about it and I finally decided to try some to see for myself. In my opinion, there's no comparison between raw milk and what most Americans drink! Once I had raw milk in me, I tasted the difference and I could feel the difference. My nails were stronger from the raw milk. This is when I started paying attention and learning about what Sam Biser's book Resurrection calls "the blessings of the barn yard."

At that same time, I was doing colonics every single week, but it wasn't improving my health to the level I still hoped I could attain. It seemed as if everything I ate caused an allergic reaction. Even eating broccoli increased the numbness in my hand. I began to have visions of myself being allergic to everything and living like young David Vetter, the "boy in the bubble" depicted in that John Travolta movie!

I realized it might be time to start working on parasites. I tried different formulas to kill parasites and immediately saw "ascari" come out—little bits of stuff that looks like rice. Dr. Hulda Clark has an extensive protocol on killing parasites that I began to follow. I even took her diagram to make my own "zapper," a device designed to put a mild electric current through one's body.

I was willing to try anything at that point, no matter how odd it seemed. The name sounded worrisome, like I was going to "get zapped" and my hair would fly every which way, but it turned out to be a very low current, one that I couldn't really even feel. She recommends that you make your own, and she gives the instructions and lists all of the materials you need to buy from a store, like Radio Shack. When I went to the store, the clerk looked over my list of supplies and blurted out, "It looks like you're making a vibrator here!" I tried to explain to him, "No, I was making a 'Zapper'." Right in the middle of trying to describe a Zapper (which was just digging the hole deeper) I realized the impossibility of trying to fix the situation. Sometimes we just have to suck it up and ride it out. This was one of those times. So, with a slightly crimson face I paid for my materials and walked out, with my head held up.

Once home with the supplies, I tried to follow the instructions for making my own Zapper but it was a crazy mess and never seemed quite right. Eventually, I simply ended up buying a commercial Zapper instead of trying to make own. The current was not as strong as I expected. The device might have been doing something to me but I didn't feel it at the time. I continued to use the Zapper, following her instructions, willing to try it so I could get healthy again.

Stressful Blessings

I was getting more and more ill, afraid of not being able to ever fully heal. It's a long story, but I believe it bears relating here.

It was the 4th of July, 2004 and I was getting increasingly ill. I had been going through a tremendous bout of stress and had some serious self-esteem issues. This will become more apparent as the story unfolds.

We wanted to do something nice for my husband's grandmother, to whom he had been very close. She was disabled and living in a skilled-care facility where she couldn't get out much. We decided to rent a handicapped-fitted van and take her out for her birthday to watch fireworks. It was going to be a jolly time for us all and we were really looking forward to it.

I was on my way back home after going to a neighboring city to rent the specialized van. I was driving the van, my husband and son joining me for the impromptu road trip, when a cloudburst released a torrent of rain, flooding the highway. Despite my terrified efforts, the van was out of control; it slid off the road and into a gully. I looked out the window and saw the water was all the way up to the driver's-side door handle! The van was filling up with water and my son was screaming. I cried out, "Oh my GOD!" And, just like that, the water receded as quickly as it had been coming in. The van started right up, and we got out of that jam intact and unharmed. Still, it spooked me! When I was forced off the Interstate and into that gully filled with water, it was only by the grace of God the van didn't tip over as it plunged downwards.

I had already been struggling with issues concerning how people felt about me. The van incident was the proverbial straw that broke the camel's back. It just felt like the whole world hated me. Even when I was trying so hard to do something good by taking grandma out for the day, something terrible happened to me.

I had a lot of drama-trauma in my life: my husband and I had a couple of extreme marital problems and low self-esteem issues were weighing so heavy on me that I had almost given up. Now, I can see that everything I went through was a huge blessing, a catalyst for the changes I needed to make to be who I finally am today.

I always just wanted people to like me, and I tended to blame myself for anything that happened. I thought that I had caused all the bad things to happen, that I had done something wrong in my marriage. I was ignoring the fact that it does take two in any relationship! After a period of time, it all took its toll. When I consider that I lived this trauma day after day, month after month, year after year, I realize now that I had lost my sense of self.

I had even consulted the pastor of my church during the second bout of marital issues, and he suggested a book called Battlefield of the Mind by Joyce Meyers. It states that when things like that go on in your head for a long period of years, Satan is taking over and playing tricks in your head, bringing you to a point where you don't feel loved, not even by yourself.

I was in a downward spiral: why did I try so hard when everything seemed to always go wrong? I just couldn't get out of that emotional rut. I started to eat, stuffing everything I possibly could into my mouth. It was as though I were trying to commit suicide with chocolate—a chocolate weapon. I remember going to Walgreens on the night after we'd dropped off Greg's grandmother and buying bags and bags of Hershey's and Snickers. Whatever I could find. Then I sat there, eating and eating it, along with a pie we'd bought that same night at Village Inn. Everybody had some but I finished off the pie myself!

In the days that followed, I was shoving bread, cookies, anything I could find down my throat. It was as if I wanted to get sick. And every time I'd try to start a fast — because I knew I was making myself really ill — I'd stay on it for maybe two days at a time and then quit. I would fast, quit, go back to eating, fast some more, quit, and go back to eating. I couldn't break out of it.

I started taking a lot of herbal laxatives at this time, because I couldn't GO, either. For six days following my "sugar-suicide attempt" after the accident, I did not have a single bowel movement. I began to have cartoon-like visions of my innards swarming with parasites that were feeding off all the food I had eaten since that fateful Fourth of July. It was a regular parasite Mardi Gras in there!

When I was finally able to go to the bathroom, it was as though the parasites became enraged that all the goodies were leaving. Symptoms, one after the other, started hitting me. I would begin a fast, not be able to hang on, and the whole hideous cycle then continued, day after day, and within a month, it all came to a head.

I'll never forget it. It was the day my son was starting basketball camp at Creighton University, and we were walking quite a ways across that campus from the car to his meeting place. I wasn't feeling right. It progressed with each step and I realized there was something distinctively WRONG with my feet: the numbness was back with a vengeance. In fact, it was all over my body, but especially my feet. Every inch of my skin was becoming numb from my forehead to my toes, with the only strange exception of my right thumb. Although I had no feeling left on the outside of my body, I sure could still feel the inside and it became insanely painful to walk. Every time I took a step, it felt as if broken glass was underneath my skin!

On that day, I knew my back was against the wall. Get serious about being healthy or become invalid.

CHAPTER 3

My 37 Day Fast

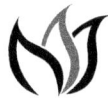

Remember the "swamp water" live juice fast? I started there. Although I enjoyed the great tasting fasts with a variety of juices, I finally realized I couldn't make everything taste good. It was time to do the thing I didn't like, because the alternatives just didn't work.

Through reading and research, I came to realize that Candida (overgrowth of yeast) and parasites played a huge role in my poor health and MS symptoms. I discovered the most effective way to kill off the overgrowth was to omit as many carbohydrates as possible.

I also realized I needed to incorporate another protocol to the fasting, which was cleansing with herbs. Inspired by Sam Biser's books, my father had been making his own concoction of herbal remedies. This peaked my interest to do the same. I then became a kitchen chemist!

I had a mixture of fine powdered herbs flying all over the house and through the vents. My son, several rooms away, would sneeze profusely from the formulas I mixed up. I found it rewarding to have the ability to create my very own medicine. This was a good thing as I needed so much with the prolonged fasting and repeated organ detoxification regimens.

This was the beginning of my journey to becoming a Master Herbalist. At first I made the products just for myself. Now, I have a full line of holistic healing supplements. The ones I used for this 37 day fast were: PowerPoop, PowerGrab, CayennePower, DetoxPower Tea, EchinaceaPower, KidneyPower, and LiverPower. You will find a complete list of all the products I carry in Appendix A. If you are more a do-it-yourself type, in Chapter 19 I share how to make your own tinctures, teas, and encapsulations. It is easy to make your own medicine and you too can become a kitchen chemist.

Parasites, PowerGrab, and PowerPoop

I decided to cleanse out my organs, something I had never given credence to before. Now I realize just what the advocates mean about the importance of including organ cleansing as part of the healing process. This is when I began using my PowerGrab and PowerPoop Intestinal Formulas to grab stuff from my colon's walls.

It had been five days on this fast, and I wasn't really seeing much improvement when usually I would see some improvement in one or two days. I was finally off the rollercoaster of fasting and binging, and was doing everything right. I couldn't understand why it didn't seem to be working.

It was the sixth day of the fast and it happened to be a Saturday. I decided that I would consume just water and the protocol of herbs. I began to feel better immediately! So I kept doing water, hoping I could last until the following Tuesday when I was slated to go back to work. I assumed that, by then, I'd be running out of energy.

But it was the exact opposite.

My energy was good and getting better by the day. I decided, "Heck, I'm not going to fix what isn't broken," so I just kept at it, with water and herbs only, for a full ten days. Every single day I felt like I was getting more relief. After ten days on just water, Day 16, and I began to feel my energy running low again. I followed my intuition to add the live juice back into my fasting regime.

At this point I knew I should stick to pure greens in the live juice. My body was undergoing significant changes as it healed. I decided to not make it complicated — stick to one vegetable and see what happens.

So I picked just one: the cucumber. Why did I choose cucumber juice? Cucumbers are very palatable vegetables for live juicing, a good source of potassium, and low in carbohydrates. I would also add a splash of sea salt to the mix, as it is rich in trace minerals. Plus, once I added the pinch of sea salt it diminished some of the old symptoms that were returning. My body needed it.

The results ended up being phenomenal.

Also, I took PowerGrab Intestinal Formula, Monday thru Friday, and the PowerPoop at night to get everything pushed through. Every Saturday, prior to the liver flush I juiced one bulb of garlic (approximately 25 cloves), which made about one ounce of garlic juice. When I drank that shot of garlic juice, it burnt like the devil from my throat to my chest but, beyond that, I couldn't feel a thing.

Remember those parasites?

After consuming the garlic juice the first couple of Saturday's, I could feel something moving from finger to finger and back and forth. It was like the parasites were moving under my skin — I could literally feel it. I thought I'd even be able to see it happening, but that was not the case. I could sure feel it, though!

The garlic juice stirred up those parasites and ultra-stimulated the liver. Which made the liver flush even more powerful. The new routine was followed by a colonic every Sunday, plus following Dr. Hulda Clark's parasite protocol. I was drinking a gallon, if not more of water every day (distilled is the best choice) and adding in herbal teas, as well.

If all of this sounds eccentric of me, I felt that I had to get a little eccentric — I was that sick! I was working on the colon Monday through Friday, and on Saturdays I would do the liver flush. I repeated that, every single week, throughout the thirty-seven-day fast. I continued working on my kidneys too, simply by drinking lemon water and cayenne. Because I was in so much pain it was easy to stay disciplined and on track.

Story Worth Repeating

I was also taking a nutrition class at this time, one where the teacher was fond of telling us to be extra-careful when doing liver flushes. I thought, "Oh boy, lady, you don't want to know what I'm doing every single Saturday, along with this fast!" I was paying close attention to my body and following my intuition as to what was best for me at the time.

My health was in critical condition. I knew this intensive routine was what I needed and would pump things up a notch and I am glad I didn't follow her advice.

Rock Salts Rocked!

One day during this treatment cycle, I was just home after another trip to the health food store picking up some rock salt for my salt grinder. Remembering how adding a little salt in the cucumber juice made the tingling sensation I had been experiencing go away, I knew the minerals from salt had great benefit to my body. When filling up the salt grinder, suddenly something urged me to throw some of it in my mouth. I felt possessed, and kept going back for more and more until I had consumed between a quarter to half a cup of salt.

Since just after the start of the fast, I had been feeling something in my colon moving up and down. It even felt like some of it was already hanging out! I got a mirror to check, but couldn't see a thing. It felt like it was on some sort of weird elevator inside me, going up almost all the way to the top of my butt crack and then back down again. Up and down. It wouldn't travel fast; it was actually moving quite slowly. I asked the person doing my colonics if she could see anything, but she didn't.

After consuming the large amount of rock salt earlier in the day, I did my usual Saturday evening liver flush before bedtime. I woke up that night at about one in the morning really needing to go to the bathroom. I turned on the bathroom light because, by then, I was curious and wanted to see what would come out of me. From the liver flush, I expected to see stones. But instead, there was this thing in the toilet — a CREATURE the size and look of a sunny-side up egg, but instead of it being yellow where the yolk would be, it was a reddish pink. I thought, "Oh my Lord, that lady was right!! There's a chunk of my liver there, floating in the toilet." I had no idea what this thing was.

Because by now I was wide-awake, I went down to the computer and checked emails. There was an email from www.CureZone.com, and the person who had written it said that she, too, felt something crawling under her skin. Someone had replied and said, "Well, it is parasites," and because she had given her website to check out parasite pictures, I went to that site and found it. That thing floating in my toilet was one of the 25 pictures of parasites!

The coincidence just blew me away.

I realized what I saw in the toilet and had felt moving around in my rectum was the parasite, not a chunk of my liver. In reading the website and theories on parasites, I discovered that parasites will multiply, out of control, when a person has a lack of salt intake. Salts keep them in check. That huge intake of salt I gobbled down combined with the herbal supplements and fasting was evidently what finally killed the creature and got it out of me. And yes, after that, the feeling of something moving in my rectum was GONE.

Remember the section Story Worth Repeating of the person who said to be so cautious about liver cleansing? Let this be a tremendous lesson: I learned that if you go half way then you will get half the healing. I am so glad that I followed my intuition on what was right for my body. I had to pump it up, be disciplined and committed; otherwise I would have never received the health I did. So, do not be afraid, you may have to do the same. Go all the way. Do not stop.

As for those liver flushes, I had good results. I passed stones anywhere from the size of sand to the size of my thumbnail — that's big! And, although I did not have high cholesterol, I could see I passed cholesterol stones too. They are easy to identify because they are generally greenish.

Many of these results didn't start happening until Day Sixteen, but from then until Day Thirty-Seven, they were remarkable!

The Unexpected

I must give credit to my PowerGrab Intestinal Formula here. It is my favorite formula. Starting on Day 16, I began the elimination of approximately 14 feet of hard casing from the intestinal walls. Dry, hard, solid, and crumbly sludge exited my body. The hard casing was like the inside of an old rotted pipe in your house, filled with calcium, minerals, and other debris from years of use. When I was getting the colonics, the practitioner administering them could hardly believe it! She had been seeing me weekly, and sharing my results every step of the way, but even she was shocked when what the colonics was pulling out of me shot through her machine, hitting the pipe and dinging it! I knew it was hard and dry because, when I would go to wipe my rear in the bathroom, it was dry and crumbly. I thought that was the oddest thing.

And how did I know it was fourteen feet? Because every time it would come out, it was anywhere from twelve to eighteen inches long, and this went on from Day Sixteen to Day Thirty-Seven. Granted, it took some time for the PowerGrab to do the job. What it does is grab the old fecal matter that's been there for years. It's stuff that you could have eaten when you were a kid, an old turkey sandwich in there since you were 10 years old! Everything we've eaten has the potential to have gotten stuck in our colons, building up a casing on the small and large intestinal walls. The PowerGrab formula, however, coats the stuff, softens it up, and grabs it. The process is very soothing to the lining, and it helps heal the holes in your gut and intestines. Think of this as sort of putting "your poop in a group," and then easily eliminating it!

Final Week

Always listen to your intuition.

All the symptoms I suffered from 30 days ago was just about to the finish line of healing, and I can remember that the final straw. I was going up a short set of stairs at home and I was experiencing it took everything I had to climb seven steps of stairs. My energy was at an all time low.

This is where I now understood when so many talked about a 30 day cleanse, rather than the 37-day fasting I did. The last week my energy levels were on a teeter-totter. It would go up then down, getting harder to hold on to the fast each day of that last week. Through the complete fasting, I had never experienced this until the last week.

Truth be told; I wanted to make it to forty days, like Jesus, had done. I could not do so. I had to admit, "Gina is Gina and Jesus was Jesus" and be happy with thirty-seven.

Second Conclusion

The findings point to this: there's essentially a balance "from your hooter to your tooter," and diseases start from the gut. When our intestines are covered in sludge we only receive a small portion—3% to 5%—of the nutrients in what we eat. Nutrients cannot penetrate the wall of sludge. No wonder we feel poorly — we are not absorbing what we're consuming. Once the colon is clean and healthy again, we can absorb 40 - 45%!

All this requires is keeping your eyes on the prize. Initially, I kept ignoring the tap on my shoulder telling me people could heal themselves. I needed, it seems, a two-by-four clubbed over my head!

When I finally began that fast, after the numbness has spread throughout my entire body, I was ready and committed to maintaining, until I was well again. Dr. Christopher said, "Cleanse, Nourish and Heal." Although I had dabbled with fasting, I'd never gotten to true cleansing until I completed the 37-day fast. The duration is different for every person. Pay close attention to your body and follow your intuition.

If, in the end, you are asking yourself what my motivation was to try and stick with alternative practices?

The answer is easy, and I hope, self-evident: I saw tangible results that altogether changed my outlook on disease and restored me to a state of good health, vitality, and optimism. Do not take my word for it, try it yourself; you will be glad you did!

CHAPTER 4

THE FINAL BIT OF HEALING

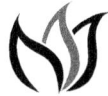

On the day the fast ended, nearly all the symptoms were gone. I still had discomfort in my feet. It felt like two golf balls were stuck in the balls of my feet. I expected healing would be gradual throughout the fast, but that by the end of it I would be completely healed. So when I had to end the fast but was not completely healed, I thought, "Okay, I can eat for a couple of weeks, and before I take a turn for the worse, I'll return to the fast." I thought I'd build up the nutrition in my body and then start another fast. Instead, I continued to eat and even started getting a little cocky with my eating habits. I had stayed away from wheat and gluten, but now I started adding them back: I had a piece of toast, and it had been years since I had toast.

The balls on the bottom of my feet continued to shrink. I even had some broccoli, something that I was so sure that I had been allergic to in the past, and the balls on my feet kept shrinking more and more. My colon got so much better that, within a couple of weeks, when I thought I was going to have to start another fast, those balls on the bottom of my feet were completely gone. To paraphrase Dr. Christopher, a world-renowned herbalist, "When you're allergic to different food items, you need cleanse your body, to rid yourself of the allergies."

Taking my cue from this, I began to add back in all the foods I was heretofore "allergic" to, and I continued to heal once my body was cleansed. That's when I understood more than ever the allergies to food theory. I had given my colon enough stimuli in those thirty-seven days for it to work and work really well!

I would eat...and I would have to poop. I would wake up...and have to poop. Do any form of exercise...and have to poop. It was great. I can't even remember a time when my colon worked like that. That is how it is supposed to work: you should be going three times a day, with stools a little bigger around than several pencils.

My Toxic Work Environment

Looking back, I now realize that getting all the chemicals from my line of work out of me was a key, too. On a daily basis I had been breathing harmful fumes and absorbing toxins through my skin while I was doing nails. Most men would walk into the nail salon and say, "Wow, the smell is horrendous!" This should have been a clue, but I, like most women, have been taught to ignore the smell. Bad tastes and smells are warning signals that something is hazardous for us. We ignore these warnings at the peril of our own health.

Were chemicals what caused the MS?

No. My father has symptoms of MS and his mother who was diagnosed with MS, were never sitting in nail salons. The chemicals were just one piece of the pie; it always takes several pieces to make a whole one. So, even if some of it was the chemicals, genetic predisposition to the disease and poor nutrition were equally influential factors.

Not long after I closed my shop in 2005, the numbness in my fingertips spread up my arm. I had eliminated all of the offending food groups, deleting wheat and gluten and even meat at one time, plus all the detoxing and fasting. But I had never removed myself from the chemicals. I did a short fast that summer. Now that I was away from all the chemicals I achieved that final level of healing which at last cleared away all the numbness in my body. I have been symptom free since then, and it was four years in July 2009.

Dreams Happened

I was beginning to find the blessings from all the personal challenges in my life.

One day at church, the pastor, whom I had considered to be my very good friend and ally, wouldn't even look at me. I concluded that really he just hated me. I even got up and left the service. Really, it was all created in my mind. Eventually, I stopped to consider that he had other people in church that day to deal with, not just me.

From that time on, it really hit me hard: people did not hate me—in fact, they really like me! It was everything I'd been living with daily that caused me to practically lose my mind. I began to focus on what I could do for myself and how I could stop cutting myself down. I began to see my own self-worth again. If that hadn't happened, I don't think I could have changed my mental attitude or situation.

My sense self-worth began to come back. Once that started, I realized that I needed to follow my dreams and my path. My path was becoming a Master Herbalist. I couldn't find anyone locally that could help to achieve the healing like, the other Master Herbalist I read about. Therefore, I attended Dr. Christopher's school (who is deceased but his wonderful kids still run the program) in Springville, Utah. This is the same program Dr. Schulze attended. I got to meet the very people I'd heard about, read about, seen on tapes, and heard on the radio. Now I've completed my master herbalist course, I can say without reservation it was an awesome experience

All of these people are mentors to me, and I am deeply grateful for their work. I now know that everything that happened to me has happened for a reason. I am living my life's dream now to help and inspire people to take control of their health. The even greater blessing is that I really believe that all of this happened to me so that I would be able to teach and pass my knowledge along…to you. What a great feeling — there is nothing like it.

It has all come to fruition, along with the creation of my two websites, www.gina-kopera.com and my store at www.ginascorner.com.

Spiritual Inspiration When I Needed It Most

It was after my very first "unintentional" fast in April of 2000. About six months after that fast, I received a box from United Design, a distributor of picture frames that I sold in the gift-shop part of my salon. I got a box and didn't know where it came from because I hadn't been ordering anything. It struck me as strange that the shipping container had my street address but the invoice was addressed to the Garden of Gods. What are the chances of that, in this computer age?

Inside was a beautiful cross. I called them and reported the mistake. They told me to just donate it to some non-profit and they'd reship to the right business. When I got off the phone an odd thing hit me: had I been actually buying a cross, it probably would have been that exact one. When I thought harder about all this, it seemed like it wasn't a mistake, like it had been meant for me as an inspiration to help others who wanted to help themselves!

Everything I describe here really has a basis in the Bible: the fasting, the herbs, the juicing, the fruits, vegetables and greens—you can find it all, the whole journey, in scripture. This journey had come to me, not with a tap on the shoulder, but with a two-by-four over the head!

The story does not end here. During this time, my son was ill as well. Because of what I went through, I was able to give him back a healthy life. I applied some of these same natural healing techniques to give him a life free of pharmaceutical medications.

CHAPTER 5

CURING MY SON TOO

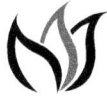

During my 37 day fast, another crisis happened. Devin, our son, got sick — really sick. He was only 8 years old. I had commented to my husband that we needed to stop letting him eat junk food and sugar. I didn't want him to follow down the same path of poor health from bad dietary habits. For example, I had noticed he had the same bumps on his arms I used to have, the ones which disappeared during my non-intentional fast. I was worried he inherited a genetic curse from me.

The Symptoms

I got a call from the daycare that something was wrong with Devin. They couldn't figure out what was going on. Apparently, he was a little limp and he was saying things that didn't make sense, so I had them put him on the phone. I asked him what the matter was, and he answered me in gibberish, like he was drunk. The daycare worker told me they were taking him to the hospital.

I was with a client at the time, said I had to leave, and drove as fast as I could to be there. On the way, I called my husband to have him go to the hospital; he was closer than I was. Greg got there just as Devin arrived, and when Greg pulled him out of the van, he was stiff and staring into space. This was a complete shock:

just hours ago we had a totally functioning, normal child and now, dramatically, everything had changed.

By the time I got to the ER, Devin was on a bed with everyone standing around him, crying. He was still not making sense and was staring into space, his hands formed into fists and his body rigid. I thought to myself, "Gina, with everything YOU'VE read, what you can do?" And it came to me: the bottom line with any illness is dehydration of the body, so I thought to start with water. I went and asked one of the nurses for a little cup so I could give him some, and she said, "No." They said he didn't need it because he would throw it up. I felt the anger rise up in me; I hadn't asked them if I could give him chocolate malt from Dairy Queen or anything—just water! When they saw me getting angrier by the moment, they finally relented and gave me a cup.

I filled it with maybe a scant ounce of water—after all, he wasn't functioning and it wasn't as though he could have gulped it down. Gently, I coaxed him to drink these couple of sips. With just that little bit of water, he said a word, a normal word that wasn't jumbled up!

I helped him with two more ounces of water, reassuring him, "Devin, I'm going to help you. Have just a little more water." Even that small amount of water so revived that he took the cup from me, crushed it up, and said a couple more words. I remember thinking, "Oh God, it's working! This is unbelievable!" (Note: Everybody, remember to feed your body water!)

Next, they prepped him for a CT scan. My husband carried him to the X-ray room and Devin did throw up all over the place. After that, he was brought back to the ER where they finally put him on an IV of saline solution: water and salt. I'll tell you right now: the moment that went into his veins, he uttered the first normal sentence he'd said since this whole episode began. That's the power of water.

Following Conventional Medicine

Within a few weeks, the diagnosis was in: epilepsy. My husband and I began to discuss treatment options for him. We were of differing opinions. My husband wanted to follow conventional medicine practices; I was convinced nutrition and holistic healing techniques were the best option. I wasn't talking about putting my little boy on a fast, but there were lots of kid-friendly ways that I could treat him "my way." What I did on the fast could also be obtained by eating a mucous-free diet, but it did require an extended commitment to the program.

I just knew if I put Devin on a healthy diet, everything could start changing. My husband agreed to it, with the following caveat: "We'll follow it your way UNLESS and UNTIL he has one more seizure — then he goes on the meds." I agreed to this, confident if I put him on a ketogenic diet, and a protocol of no sugar and lots of water, it would work.

The ketogenic diet was developed at Johns Hopkins University for use in treating epilepsy in children. It is the Atkins Diet "Plus." It has extremely low carbs - no sugar at all, nothing in the way of fruit or juices—what everyone loves. They even want the kids to drink cream on that diet.

I didn't go to that extreme, but it was pretty much meat, vegetables, and more meat. Milk was okay if it contained the higher percentage of milk fat. At that time I had already introduced the raw milk, which was even better for him. We stayed on that protocol and it was working great for his health. But I'll tell you, it was a hair-pulling experience. I even offered Devin the deal that if anyone gave him anything sugary or any candy, I would buy it from him. This was a moneymaking deal for him!

We had really good results for about three weeks with the ketogenic diet, but you don't always have total control over what other people will feed your kid. People put sugar in many foods that you wouldn't call particularly "sweets," and they think to themselves, "Oh, this isn't going to hurt him," but of course, it does. He had another seizure, and I abided by my word: he went on anti-seizure drugs. I was ready to tear my hair out with frustration. It felt like the whole world was against my efforts. I was hitting my limits and then some!

I went to visit a friend in Chicago for a little break and to get some perspective. On my trip, I was listening to Wayne Dyer tapes. Dyer is a motivational speaker who is absolutely wonderful. He was talking about the experience of receiving healing from a kahuna practitioner. Dyer explains that until you've had "conscious contact" with this type of healing, you cannot know it. It's just like you can't read about swimming and then know how to swim: you've got to get into the water and DO it. (And for all of you reading this, it's the same thing: you can't just follow what I'm saying without trying it for yourself and actually experiencing the type of healing I'm describing.)

So, Devin was on Depakote. He wasn't having any more seizures, but then we didn't have our same kid, either! He would become incredibly tired and had no energy at all. He seemed like a zombie. It was the saddest thing.

It was at this point a client of mine recommended a movie she had seen on the Lifetime channel, "First, Do No Harm," starring Meryl Streep. In the movie, her son had epilepsy. She kept searching for a way to heal her son from the serious seizures, and she was heading right for the poor house, going the traditional medical route. Willing to explore all healing options she came across the same ketogenic diet that I had tried on my son! It even shows Meryl Streep's character taking her son to Johns Hopkins, going through hell and high water, jumping through hoops to get him there because other medical professionals were telling her there was no scientific proof that it would work (just like had happened with me).

After I saw that film, I asked Devin's doctor about this diet, and she sniffed at me, "if he eats just one M&M on that diet, it will negate all the rest of the results and it will be ruined." I persisted, "What's your point? Wouldn't you try everything, if it were your kid?" I was convinced parasites were part of the problem. She told me there were only about five parasites that would be able to make it all the way up to the brain. That was five more than I wanted in Devin's system.

I couldn't find support anywhere for my ideas. I gave up using my techniques on him and tried to be as supportive as I could. The stress was making me more ill than my original sickness had made me!

Eventually, I let them go ahead with the traditional medical tests EEG and MRI. The EEG was pretty painless, but to do the MRI, they had to inject dye into his veins. The first time, the nurse missed his vein. When she tried to do it the second time, my little child turned into something akin to the Incredible Hulk; they could hardly hold him down, he was so mad. You can't blame him, it hurts. So that's when I told them, "This is enough. If you can't do the MRI without dye, then you're not going to do it." It was heartbreaking to see him in such agony.

Changing to Holistic Healing

By March of 2005, I closed down my shop. The plan was to be home looking after Devin and helping my husband run his construction business. Devin was supposed to be on Depakote full time, but he was inconsistent. He'd take it one day and not take it the next. My child, once active and vibrant, was now lifeless and lethargic from the Depakote. I kept silent, but continued personal research into healing epilepsy naturally so that, if anything did happen, I could be helpful.

Greg finally said, "You know what? Why don't we just try going without the drug and doing it your way, and see what happens." Seeing our child, who had always been so full of life, become a walking zombie was something we just couldn't stand. I was thrilled with the change, and now that I was home full-time, I was able to monitor his diet better and give Devin better foods. Everything I tried would help a little, but it was after liver flushes and focusing on cleansing the colon and the kidneys that the seizures reduced in frequency. The seizures were happening about once every three weeks. He'd either have a seizure or a headache. At the beginning of my treating him, I just couldn't seem to get past that. Eventually, I found out certain parasites will re-hatch every three weeks which was why these seizures kept coming like clockwork. That's when I started to follow the parasite protocol of Dr. Hulda Clark.

But I did get one scare! Right in the middle of this process, Devin, now 9, had the biggest seizure I had ever seen. We were in the car on the interstate, and I realized that he was having a seizure. Here I was, on the highway, and he was leaning, about to topple over onto me, with his face turning blue! I just headed for the hospital; I didn't know what else to do, at that moment.

Now, looking back on it, I understand that when he was leaning toward me his tongue was dropping back, suffocating him. At the time I instinctually pushed him forward; once I did that, he started breathing easily again and coming around. We went back home instead of the hospital. He got out of the car — it was like looking at a drunken person — but he went to bed and he was fine. Still, I knew he'd had a grand mal seizure. It scared the daylights out of me.

I started to second-guess whether I was hurting him with my methods, but everything I did spread all his symptoms farther apart. With all that I know now, I can surmise was that his body was trying to kill off some of the big parasites.

Once we did the parasite treatment, things really started to improve. Prior to that, we made sure the colon was working (since pooping is very important), and we did a liver flush—made kid-friendly, of course. I put the olive oil and Epsom salts that he needed for the flush into capsules. He was so good to cooperate with me; especially after having been on those drugs which he hated so. We were a sight to see, both of us in bed with castor oil packs on our liver and heating pads.

That night I made lemonade popsicles from lemon, stevia (a natural sweetener) and water—he loved those. He got that instead of dinner on the night of the flush (plus his last meal for lunch was always his choice of where to go). Sure enough, he had liver stones coming out until four o'clock the next day. It was unbelievable. A nine-year-old kid!

Devin had done many of my treatments: colon and liver flush, lemon water for the kidneys, tinctures, and capsules. After the parasite elimination, he went five or six months between seizures, but he was still having occasional headaches; I just couldn't get him to the finish line (like I couldn't get rid of that small bit of residual numbness with myself at one time).

The Final Step

His last seizure was that following autumn, August of 2005. He had a seizure the first day of fifth grade and missed his first day of school. I had recently read Sam Biser's book, Resurrection, and the first chapter of that book summarized all my thoughts: using a wider selection of vegetables, adding in more meat, and drinking raw milk. Then it hit me: Sam talks of the "blessings of the barnyard" and the power of protein. When I first had Devin on the ketogenic diet, his body responded really well. Devin's colon worked great and his energy level was great. He is also a carb junkie — he loves sugar, pasta, breads and all that, as do most Americans — and I realized he hadn't been getting much protein recently. Bisers' protein shake recipe offers a really high source of protein—raw milk and organic farm-fresh eggs. I thought, "I've been doing a shake with Devin that did use raw milk. I used it with the Cookies and Cream flavor of Spiru-Tein (a soy protein powder) that he liked. I think I'll throw in some raw eggs."

So I made one up, blended it a bit, took a drink of it myself to make sure no one was going to keel over from it, and gave it to him! He drank it and from that day on, he did not have seizures. I even got away with the raw egg bit for a while, until he caught on to what I was doing.

Other Master Herbalist say, when the body seizes it is searching for missing nutrients. In Devin's case, it definitely was the protein from the raw egg and whatever else those shakes had to offer him. This was the final addition that Devin's nutrition needed in order to clear up his symptoms once and for all. Thank you, Sam Biser, for showing me how to take him to the finish line!

Devin was well again. We were good about it at the start: a shake every day. Then symptoms were gone and it was so easy to forget about it. The frequency dropped to every other day, then once a week, until they slipped out of the routine entirely. Eventually poor eating habits caught up with him again, and in January 2009 Devin had another seizure. I felt terrible that I let him get ill again. But, picking back up with the nutritional foods again did the trick and we are better disciplined now. He's well again. That was just a reminder. Any of us can slip off the path, even me, who knows it and lives it, but it is just a slip. Returning to the foods and holistic practices that keep us healthy is easy to do.

YOUR BODY, FOOD, AND HEALTH

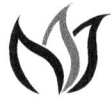

Chapter 6

There Is a Problem, but There Is a Solution!

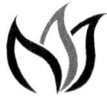

Ninety percent of all diseases have a starting point in the colon, liver, or both. Supreme cleanliness is the first step towards a healthy, powerful body. Any retention of morbid matter or waste of any kind will retard your progress toward recovery. These organs are no different than the filters in your car. Would you get a new car and never change the oil? I think not! Just like maintaining your car, your organs need to be flushed out.

Originally, I didn't put much merit in cleansing out the organs. The first time, with my non-intentional fast, I wasn't cleansing out a thing. Even though I got totally healed, it didn't last, and the symptoms returned with a vengeance. I don't want you to go through years of ups and downs, the way I did, before grasping importance of cleansing the organs.

How long will this take? It varies by individual, but remember the current condition of your body didn't happen in one day, and just one day isn't going to complete your cleansing process, either. Also, this is not a one-time process. Maintaining your health means following regular cleansing protocols and proper nutrition.

I just want to put in this note, that merely taking milk thistle or some herbal combination for the liver or 20 liver flushes is helpful but will not take you to the finish line. Taking an herbal supplement to get you colon moving is helpful but will not take you to the finish line. This entire protocol will explain in detail what you must do, to complete every piece of the pie, which is a must to allow your body to work in harmony.

The Good News

Sometimes, when life presents us with challenges that seem unfair or unsolvable, it gives us an opportunity to grow in our search for solutions. We can't learn anything from experiences we're not having! Consider them your greatest blessing, even though it may not feel like it at the time. This journey is an ongoing work in progress.

There are still things that I need to conquer. What I have found to be really helpful in this journey are books and CD's of motivational and inspirational speakers that help give guidance on positive thinking.

I was raised to believe that if there's a problem, there's a solution. I am going to share with you the solution that I experienced one that can possibly save your life, just as it has saved mine. This type of healing goes under a pretty simple theory:

Cleanse, nourish, and let thy body heal itself

During my four years of fasting protocols, I wish I had the personal guidance and support of what I am here to offer you. The time, effort, frustration, and cost of going through this journey alone would have been greatly reduced.

Empower Yourself

We've all heard it said, "Knowledge is Power." There are things that are good for your body and things that are bad for it. When you can identify your symptoms and learn how to rid yourself of them, you will see amazing results. It takes desire, dedication, perseverance, and keeping your eye on the prize at all times. Let's get out of being the victim and instead be the victor. What do you have to lose? Try it and see the results for yourself!

Of all the important natural healing precepts, the first is to treat those specific organs that do the body's elimination work: your bowel, liver, kidneys, blood and your largest organ, the skin. These need to be strong, toned, and functioning properly. They do the work of eliminating toxins.

There are poisons in us that must be flushed out. They will not be extracted as a part of your body's normal processes. If you try to heal before your elimination organs are ready to handle the job, the healing will likely not last.

I have an awesome vitality program for you that is quite aggressive. This is for healing from a debilitating disease or a healthy body not to get sick, and then staying well. When you are at this point, you must be more aggressive than the disease, because the most aggressive will win. Once you learn the program, you will feel empowered because you have taken control of your life, mentally and physically. You will have the knowledge that empowers you to live a great, symptom-free, healthy life, NOW!

Hippocrates (hih POK ruh teez)

Born in 460 B.C. Died in 377 B.C.

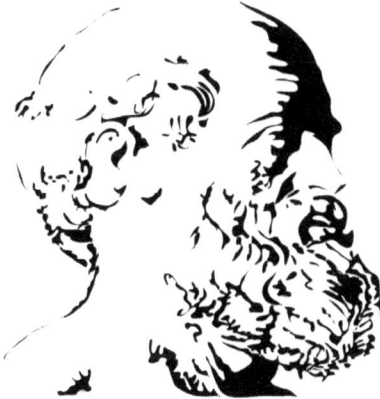

Hippocrates is history's most popular physician. What fascinates me about this man is that it has been countless centuries and his words and philosophies are still recognized to this day. He is regarded as the Father of Medicine and one of the greatest physicians of his time and best known as the author of the Hippocratic oath. For some centuries this oath used by various physicians and we continue to apply his legendary words, "First, Do No Harm."

Hippocrates was on the island of Cos, Greece. In his work, Hippocrates traveled throughout Greece practicing medicine and eventually became the founder of the Hippocratic School of Medicine. His philosophy of medicine was based on observations and in the study of the whole human body. He held the belief that illnesses had a physical and sensible explanation.

He rejected the views held by his contemporaries, who considered illnesses to be supernaturally caused or caused by demonic spirits and disfavor of the gods. Hippocrates believed the body must treat the cause, not symptom. He believed in the natural healing process for your body: quality sleep, diet, fresh air, and cleanliness. He also noted there were distinct differences in disease symptoms, and some were better able to cope with their disease and illness than others.

Let's return to the Hippocratic ideas of health, and discover again how to heal ourselves.

Get to the CAUSE not the symptom.

I have worked with clients on healing their individual bodies. They are usually puzzled at the answer I have for how to help themselves. The answer seems too simple, it almost sounds silly.

Even if your symptom is an achy foot, the key place to start your healing is (you will get tired of me saying this) your colon. Get your colon moving. Plus drink plenty of water and exercise. Simple, right? Look at the whole body and not just the pain in your foot. Your organs are all linked to ailments that you suffer. It's the cause you need to look for, not the symptom. Cleanse, nourish and let thy body heal itself. Try it!

CHAPTER 7

BODY TALK

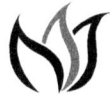

Our bodies are remarkable:

- The length of the small and large intestines averages 25 ft in an adult.

- The largest organ is your skin; it is average of 16.1-21.5 sq ft.

- The liver is the second largest internal organ in the human body, weighing three to six pounds

- The kidneys delicate tubules which run from the kidneys to the bladder could be pinched through with a fingernail!

Amazing isn't it?!

The Colon

Shown in the picture is the large intestine, extending from the cecum to the rectum. It was formerly referred to the large intestines, now it is also commonly now called the colon. The colon is a part of the digestive system, which it is a series of organs from the mouth to the anus.

Location

The large intestines otherwise known as the colon, is shaped like an inverted U. The colon has three sections and is housed within the abdominal cavity. The names of these sections are: ascending, transverse, and descending. It begins in the lower right side of the abdominal cavity, located around the waist area, and runs along the right side of the abdominal cavity, called the ascending colon, until it reaches just below the liver and stomach. Here, it crosses the abdomen vertically and is known as the transverse colon. Finally, it descends down on the left side of your abdominal cavity and is called the descending colon and continues on to its exiting point at the rectum/anus.

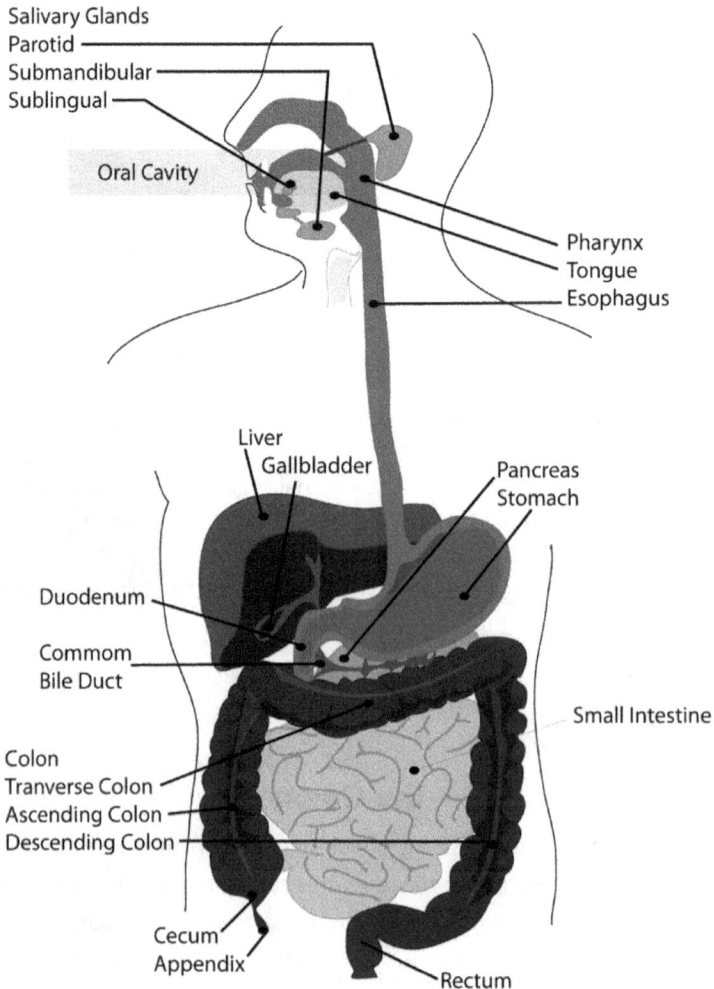

Colon Function

The colon is responsible for the finishing stages of the digestive process.

1. Absorb the remaining water and electrolytes from indigestible food matter

2. Assumes, assimilate, and stores food remains of what was not digested from the small intestines

3. Eliminates solid waste (feces)

The colon secretes a quantity of mucous, but no enzymes. Food is not digested in this organ but some water is reabsorbed, and undigested food is stored and is the beginning development of feces for elimination.

It assumes and assimilates certain vitamins, processes indigestible material, and stores the waste before it is eliminated. Within the colon, the combination with small amounts of water, fiber, and vitamins mix with mucus and the bacteria that exist in the large intestine.

As the feces make its journey through the colon, the colon lining absorbs most of the water as well as some of the vitamins and minerals that are present. Bacteria which exist in the colon will feed on the fiber and break the fiber down in order to provide nutrients to nourish the cells that cover the colon. Fiber and water is a key part of a diet geared toward the colon's long-term health. For some, water alone is a laxative.

Feces will move onwards to the descending colon, causing waste to go into the rectum. Known as peristaltic action; a wave-like motion encourages feces to approach the rectum and finally, be expelled through the anus.

Constipation

Definition: Abnormally delayed or infrequent passage of usually, dry hardened feces. Over ninety percent of all diseases and malfunctions, from babies to adults stem, from the unclean intestinal tract, constipation (constipation = crowding), with infrequent, difficult evacuation and lack of coordination in the nerve and muscle functions of the colon. After time, "you do not use the peristaltic muscle, you lose it."

Balance Out the Colon

The specialized cells of the colon and bacteria exist in a fragile balance that can easily be overthrown by food, stress, chemicals in the environment, and over-growth of yeast. If digestion and colon function is not working well, the body operates in a condition known as auto-intoxication. Meaning the body is working vig-orously to rid yourself of toxins.

When your colon cannot keep up then the toxins are getting recycled, rather than expelled. A constipated colon may be at the foundation of ailments from A to Z that has to do with your body. Here is an analogy to think about: If you had a plugged up toilet would you leave it?

Of course, not, it would stink!

That is what we do with our bodies when we are constipated. It is essential to maintain proper colon function. I cannot stress this enough; this is the num-ber one place to work on first! You will find that af-fects your body from head-to-toe, young and old, it truly does not matter. No matter how small or big the health concern is; achy foot, cold, headache or incurable disease, the first place to begin is the colon. Get to POOPING and you tell me your results!

I would like to share this testimony with you.

Testimony

An unexpected result!! My son is twelve years old, affected by a seizure disorder and has autism. I have never been able to get him toilet trained, even with the help of several professional behaviorists. Because of these issues, my son is on many prescription drugs that can't be good for him long term. He also has always suffered with gut issues and has never had a normal bowel movement. [He has undergone] two different professional events of having to clean his colon out with painful and emotional trauma for him and myself.

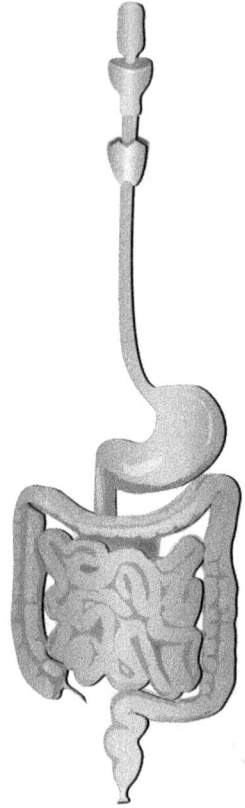

Out of pure frustration I was telling my good friend, Gina, about the ordeals and she suggested that I should try her PowerPoop to help him establish more normal looking bowels and regular movements. After five weeks on the product I got much more than I had bargained for from my son, Slader. After encouraging him for the millionth time to go poop on the toilet, this time for the very first time, Slader suddenly started walking by himself to the bathroom and I found him sitting on the toilet, having had a bowel movement!! Much to my feeling of having my own little "miracle" he has also never missed the toilet since and it has been six months for him taking the product.

His behavior has also drastically improved at school as well with no clear apparent reason other than starting the product from Gina. (He cannot speak expressively). He seems overall a more content, happier, and healthier looking boy. I am so happy to tell my story about it.

I am convinced, along with other people, about the healing effects of Gina's PowerPoop, on Slader's colon and maybe giving him the answer to an undiagnosed issue of sensory awareness with his gut!? I am very excited to continue on the venture of giving my son more of Gina's products for hopefully more continued healing to help my son.

— Sheila

The Liver

The liver is a complex organ, essential to sustaining life. Glossy in appearance, it is dark red in color from the rich supply of blood flowing through it. Your liver neutralizes harmful toxins and wastes, and stores glycogen (a blood-sugar regulator), amino acids, protein, iron, some vitamins and minerals, and fat. It produces bile that aids in digestion and regulates the levels of hormones, cholesterol, and sugars. Eventually, what we eat, drink, breathe, and absorb through our skin reaches the liver, where the nutrients are separated from the waste. This is one the liver's most critical functions. From circulation to digestion, it is continuously processing blood for use by the rest of the body.

Liver Functions (over 500!) include:

- Filtering blood
- Purifying and clearing waste products, toxins, and drugs

- Regulating and secreting substances important in maintaining your body's functions and health
- Storing important nutrients (such as glycogen glucose), vitamins, and minerals
- Metabolizing fats, proteins, carbohydrates, and hormones
- Creating bile
- Filtering internally-produced wastes and foreign chemicals
- Assimilating and storing fat-soluble vitamins
- Synthesizing blood proteins

The liver is the most durable body organ, and when the liver has moderate damage or a part of it removed, the liver can regenerate, and it may grow back to its original size. The liver has the capacity to repair itself, but even that can be exceeded by repeated or extensive damage. That means, stop doing what got you there in the first place; keep your liver healthy and cleansed as possible.

Help Your Liver Recover and Regenerate

One route you might wish to consider is liver cleansing, which the natural step is following after colon cleansing. Your body's performance will improve by cleansing and detoxing your liver. This is a powerful tool and you will see significant improvements in digestion, regularity, transit time, and augmentation of your energy levels.

Even the new laparoscopic surgical method is invasive. Surely it would be better to never have to do any surgery, instead cleaning the bile ducts naturally. Dr. Hulda Clark, author of *The Cure of All Diseases*, puts it this way, "Cleansing the liver bile ducts is the most important powerful procedure that you can do to improve your body's health." (p.553)

A liver that isn't functioning well can lead to the development of fatigue, water retention, weight gain, and many other conditions. Liver cleansing can address the serious diseases of cirrhosis and elevated enzymes of the liver or fatty liver tissue. In so doing, this saves you the expense of doctor visits or even hospital stays

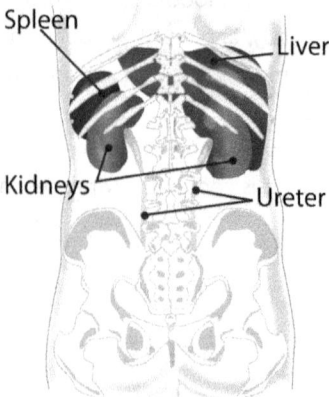
Spleen
Liver
Kidneys
Ureter

and surgery. Diet and supplements that cleanse the liver help avoid full-blown liver disease.

When blood comes to the liver free as possible of toxins, it has a much easier job of cleaning the blood. Toxins have a difficult time leaving your body after you have done a liver flush if the colon itself is blocked. It is necessary to cleanse the colon before beginning your liver cleanses.

The most rewarding flush for me was the liver flush, as the liver is the forgotten organ. Having to drink down olive oil was not my favorite pastime...until I saw the results. Then I was glad that I did!

When one is consuming olive oil by the tablespoons of 1/2 cup at a time, it does not become many people's favorite flush. When the liver is overly constipated you may experience nausea and vomiting. This may or may not happen. Do not give in now. Keep the flushes up and follow the procedure mentioned in Chapter 13. Do not miss a beat when it comes to a liver flush. Be more aggressive than your ailments or they will win. It will undoubtedly become your favorite as you receive your results.

Why is the liver so ignored?

Well, we all can feel the constipation in the colon, whereas the liver takes all kinds of abuse fairly invisibly. But when it has finally had it, and that tends to lead to serious health issues like hepatitis, cirrhosis, liver cancer, etc.

Why Liver Cleanse?

In our industrialized, developed world, we are immersed in an ocean of toxic chemicals. This is why it is crucial to cleanse your liver of the toxic waste of 21st century living.

Dr. Hulda Clark, PhD, ND, in her groundbreaking bestseller, *The Cure of All Diseases*, dramatically describes the gallstones and cholesterol that can choke the liver's biliary tubing in many people, including our children. "Imagine the situation if your garden hose had marbles in it. Much less water would flow, which in turn would decrease the ability of the hose to squirt out the marbles. With gallstones, much less cholesterol leaves the body, and cholesterol levels may rise." (p.554)

Worried about gallstones? Worry, no more. Do a liver flush.

"Gallstones, being porous, can pick up all the bacteria, cysts, viruses, and parasites that are passing through the liver. In this way, nests of infection are formed, forever supplying the body with fresh bacteria. No stomach infection such as ulcers or intestinal bloating can be cured permanently without removing these gallstones from the liver." (p.554)

If the liver becomes overworked with toxic compounds and impurities then deposits of hardened bile may become trapped. Pollutants may not be flushed out of the body and can also back up into your blood stream. A toxic liver can lead to multiple health woes, such as: severe fatigue, weight gain, or water retention.

Detoxification that targets the liver can help eliminate these unwanted toxins and enable it to function properly. A healthy liver increases your energy, improves metabolism, clears-up your skin, and helps you burn unwanted fat.

My Personal Success Story

When I initially started doing liver flushes, it made me really nauseous, as if I had too much to drink. My husband asked, "Why do you do this, if it makes you that sick?" I strongly believed it would work, so I kept pushing forward and stepped it up a notch when I got to my 37 day PowerHouse Fast. The nausea was a result of my constipated liver, and after just a few liver-flushes, the side effect subsided.

The stones that came out from my liver ranged from the size of a grain of sand to the size of grapes. It is so tough to believe that all that stuff is stuck inside and you're not feeling it. Actually, I was grateful for not feeling it.

As you know, when my son was 9 years of age, I had him follow the protocol for cleansing out his organs (in a kid – friendly way) because he was suffering from seizures. Getting creative and making it kid-friendly, I put the Epsom salts and olive oil in empty capsules, and I did all of the protocols, right along with my him.

Boy-oh-boy, we looked like quite a pair!

After consuming the olive oil, we both laid in bed with castor oil packs and heating pads — quite a sight to see. His results to this flush continued through the following day, but I didn't get to see any large stones, as he went to school that day. When he got home in the late afternoon, he was still clearing stones the size of sand grains – and this was from a nine-year-old child.

Can you believe that?

I am still amazed.

Myself, I didn't like the olive oil in a capsule because, when the capsules dissolved, it was an immediate deposit of a gunk feeling, in the gut. I definitely prefer drinking it, but do whatever's right for you, either way.

The Kidney

Main Functions

1. Separate inorganic minerals, salts, toxins, and other waste products from the blood.

2. Conserve water, salts, and electrolytes.

Kidneys are amazing organs. Inside them are millions of microscopic blood vessels that serve as filters. They are part of the urinary system and the endocrine system. They are amongst the most important internal organs in the body, responsible for filtering the blood, regulating the urinary system, producing hormones, and regulating blood pressure.

Kidneys are extremely efficient and complex organs. If you live to the age of 50-60, you have urinated enough to fill 3 semi-truckloads with urine. Sometimes this filtering system breaks down. Failing kidneys lose their power to filter out toxic waste products resulting in kidney disease.

Your Urinary System and How it Works

The organs, tubes, muscles, and nerves that function simultaneously to create, store, and carry urine make up the urinary system. The urinary system consists of the bladder, two kidneys, two sphincter muscles, and the urethra. The system works in harmony with all your organs lungs, skin, intestines, and liver.

Kidney Stones

Can kidney problems and kidney stones be overcome?

In today's society, due to the poisonous nature of our world, kidneys are generally overworked and often end up heavily infected, inflamed, with crystalline growths, or kidney stones. This is a result of inorganic foods and drinks that are filled to the brim with not-so-good merchandise such as sugar, caffeine, or alcohol, along with a lack of water.

An infected or calcified kidney sometimes manifests in lower back pains. However, because the kidneys are "silent," a person may not be aware they received a kidney problem until the kidneys are significantly diseased. Kidney stones can be extremely painful. In severe instances, a person may suddenly collapse in great pain and be rushed to the hospital, where the sole solution is surgery, potentially ending up on a dialysis machine for life. It is very important to cleanse the kidneys in order to eliminate the calcium deposits and handle unseen infections, thus preventing kidney stones.

Blood: Your River of Life

The blood is our "River of Life". The blood, just as the liver and kidneys, is rarely given a second thought until there is a problem. No matter what the disease title is, contaminations can make the body feel weakened and tired.

The poor quality foods that we put in our bodies (breads, pastries, and refined sugars) will leach out the calcium from the veins and arteries. This leads to a calcium deficiency and general feeling of weakness. The walls of our veins, arteries, and capillaries become coated with inorganic waste materials, not allowing the cell structures to be fed. This waste forms a lining just as it does in the intestine. You absorb fewer nutrients and the lining gets weaker.

When the system gets overloaded and begins to breakdown. The originally soft, pliable tissue hardens and loses elasticity. The veins are similar to a rubber hose and cannot expand or contract with ease. They will become weak, ballooned out or brittle, and then break. If the body is functioning properly and is up to a peak performance, it now has a chance to heal itself. You help it by strengthening and toning your blood, veins, and arteries.

CHAPTER 8

CANDIDA OVERGROWTH

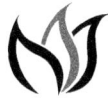

A root causes of illness, for most people, lies in the gut. You have more than 500 species of good and harmful bacteria. What causes the lack of the beneficial bacteria are high doses of antibiotics, steroids, sugar, birth control, and possibly vaccinations. Of course, some of you never took birth control (especially men — or let's hope not!). It could have been something you took years ago — 10, 20, 30, 40 years ago, etc. — that has only now started playing havoc with your digestive track. For more information of yeast in our bodies, refer to *The Yeast Connection* by William G. Crook M.D.

Candida infections are an overgrowth of yeast in the body. Symptoms run from mild to extreme. Bottom-line, if you suffer from Candida, to get rid of it you must eliminate fruits, sugar, grains, and higher carb vegetables from your diet until you get this condition under control, as these items will feed the issue. Fruits, higher carb vegetables and grains, are good for you, but also encourage overgrowth of Candida.

This is where the PowerHouse Fast Healing Program comes in, because it is quick. The Mucous-Free diet will work but will take much longer, possibly months. (That is its drawback, but it works.)

Candida is extremely difficult to get rid of, so it entirely depends on your patience, dedication, and perseverance as to what healing method will work for you. If you go the route of eating food rather than fasting out of this issue, check out online support groups, which are helpful to some.

Herbal Suggestions

Peau De Arco, an anti-fungal herb will assist in killing of the overgrowth of yeast. Sometimes capsules are not enough. A very effective way to ensure you are getting enough of Peau De Arco: make tea out of this herb as it absorbs faster to the organs and blood to help assist in the overgrowth of yeast.

  * Note: Hot tea will absorb faster than cooler tea.

Buy a pound of this herb; you're going to need it. A good source is at www.blessedherbs.com

Drink this mixture each day

- 64 ounces of water
- 1 cup of Peau De Arco
- Cover
- Let it soak for an hour
- Simmer for 20 minutes
- Let it cool
- Strain

Do this for 6 days each week for 3 weeks.

A Story Worth Sharing About The Overgrowth Of Candida

My son inherited my weak immune system, lack of digestive enzymes, and nervous system. I did not know the importance of breastfeeding and how it boosted his immune system and other health benefits. So, it was store bought formula for him.

When Devin was just six-months-old, he was given his first antibiotic for a cold - it was after that the problems began.

At six months of age, had a stuffed-up nose that would not go away. I took him to the doctor twice during this time. The first time he instructed me that it would go away, but a couple weeks later the nose issue was still there. I couldn't stand this little guy feeling this way. I insisted the doctor prescribe antibiotics for my son, as this was the only way I thought he would get better.

The doctor did give the prescription. Shortly afterwards Devin broke out in a rash all over, which was immediately followed by ear infections. Nothing seemed to help. Eventually the infections were prolonged enough the doctor decided Devin needed a tube inserted into the ear that was constantly inflamed.

Why was all this happening?! I certainly did not know then, but looking back on it today I now know these symptoms were from an overgrowth of Candida in his system. The antibiotics had killed off the good bacteria, which caused an overgrowth of the harmful bacteria. If I was faced with the same situation today, I would put:

- Couple of drops of olive oil in each ear (natural antibiotic)

- Couple drops of lobelia to help calm down the pain, and a slice of lightly baked onion (natural pain relievers)

- Garlic paste on the feet (natural antibiotic)

Candida Questionnaire

Now, to get a clear picture, fill out this questionnaire from *The Yeast Connection*. For more information get the book *The Yeast Connection* by William G. Crook, M.D. This questionnaire lists factors in your medical history that promote the growth of the common yeast, Candida Albicans (Section A), and symptoms commonly found in individuals with yeast – connected illness (Sections B and C).

Filling out and scoring this questionnaire should help you and your physician evaluate how Candida Albicans may be contributing to your health problems, but it will not provide an automatic "Yes" or "No" answer. A comprehensive history and physical examination are important. In addition, laboratory studies, x-rays, and other types of tests may also be appropriate.

Section A: History

For each "Yes" answer in Section A, circle the Point Score. Total your score, and record it at the end of the section. Then move on to Sections B and C, and score as directed.

I.	Have you taken antibiotics for acne for I month (or longer)?	50
2.	Have you, at any time in your life, taken other "broad-spectrum" antibiotics for respiratory, urinary or other infections for 2 months or longer, or for shorter periods 4 or more times in a I – year span?	50
3.	Have you taken a broad-spectrum antibiotic drug – even once?	6
4.	Have you, at any time in your life, been bothered by persistent prostatitis, vaginitis, or other problems affecting your reproductive organs?	25
5.	Have you been pregnant: 2 or more times? Pregnant I time?	5 3
6.	Have you taken birth control pills for: more than 2 years? 6 months to 2 years?	15 8
7.	Have you taken prednisone, Decadron®, or other cortisone-type drugs by mouth or inhalation** for: more than 2 weeks? 2 weeks or less?	15 6
8.	Does exposure to perfumes, insecticides, fabric shop odors, or other chemicals provoke: moderate to severe symptoms? mild symptoms?	20 5
9.	Are your symptoms worse on damp, muggy days or in moldy places?	20
10.	Have you had athlete's foot, ringworm, "jock itch" or other chronic fungus infections of the skin or nails that have been: severe or persistent? Mild or moderate?	20 10
II.	Do you crave sugar?	10
12.	Do you crave breads?	10
13.	Do you crave alcoholic beverages?	10
14.	Does tobacco smoke really bother you?	10

Total Score, Section A: _____

**The use of nasal or bronchial sprays containing cortisone and/or other steroids promotes overgrowth in the respiratory tract.

Section B: Major Symptoms

For each symptom that is present, circle the point score matching if the symptom is occasional or mild, frequent and/or moderately severe, or severe and/or disabling. Total the score for this section, and record it at the end of this section.

		occasional or mild	frequent and/or moderate	severe and/or disabling
1.	Fatigue or lethargy	3	6	9
2.	Feeling of being "drained"	3	6	9
3.	Poor memory	3	6	9
4.	Feeling "spacey" or "unreal"	3	6	9
5.	Inability to make decisions	3	6	9
6.	Numbness, burning or tingling	3	6	9
7.	Insomnia	3	6	9
8.	Muscle aches	3	6	9
9.	Muscle weakness or paralysis	3	6	9
10.	Pain and/or swelling in joints	3	6	9
11.	Abdominal pain	3	6	9
12.	Constipation	3	6	9
13.	Diarrhea	3	6	9
14.	Bloating, belching or intestinal gas	3	6	9
15.	Vaginal burning, itching or discharge	3	6	9
16.	Prostatitis	3	6	9
17.	Impotence	3	6	9
18.	Loss of sexual desire or feeling	3	6	9
19.	Endometriosis or infertility	3	6	9
20.	Cramps and/or other menstrual irregularities	3	6	9
21.	Premenstrual tension	3	6	9
22.	Attacks of anxiety or crying	3	6	9
23.	Cold hands or feet and/or chilliness	3	6	9
24.	Shaking or irritable when hungry	3	6	9

Total Score, Section B: _____

Section C: Other Symptoms:*

For each symptom that is present, circle the appropriate number in the Point Score column. Total the score for this section and record it in the box at the end of this section.

		occasional or mild	frequent and/or moderate	severe and/or disabling
1.	Drowsiness	3	6	9
2.	Irritability or jitteriness	3	6	9
3.	Lack of coordination	3	6	9
4.	Inability to concentrate	3	6	9
5.	Frequent mood swings	3	6	9
6.	Headaches	3	6	9
7.	Dizziness/loss of balance	3	6	9
8.	Pressure above ears, feeling of head swelling	3	6	9
9.	Tendency to bruise easily	3	6	9
10.	Chronic rashes or itching	3	6	9
11.	Psoriasis or recurrent hives	3	6	9
12.	Indigestion or heartburn	3	6	9
13.	Food sensitivity or intolerance	3	6	9
14.	Mucus in stools	3	6	9
15.	Rectal itching	3	6	9
16.	Dry mouth or throat	3	6	9
17.	Rash or blisters in mouth	3	6	9
18.	Bad breath	3	6	9
19.	Foot, hair or body odor not relieved by washing	3	6	9
20.	Nasal congestion or post-nasal drip	3	6	9
21.	Nasal itching	3	6	9
22.	Sore throat	3	6	9
23.	Laryngitis, loss of voice	3	6	9
24.	Cough or recurrent bronchitis	3	6	9

Total Score, Section C: _____

*While the symptoms in this section occur commonly in patients with yeast-connected illness, they also occur commonly in patients who do not have Candida.

Total Score, Section A: _____

Total Score, Section B: _____

Total Score, Section C: _____

(Add totals from Sections A, B, and C)

Grand Total: _____

Understanding Your Score

The Grand Total Score will help you and your physician decide whether your health problems are yeast-connected. Scores for women will run higher, as 7 items in this questionnaire apply exclusively to women, while only 2 apply exclusively to men.

- Yeast-connected health problems are almost certainly present in women with scores over 180, and in men with scores over 140.

- Yeast-connected health problems are probably present in women with scores over 120, and in men with scores over 90.

- Yeast-connected health problems are possibly present in women with scores over 60, and in men with scores over 40.

- With scores less than 60 for women and 40 for men, yeast is less apt to cause health problems.

Candida Questionnaire and Score Sheet excerpted from the *Yeast* Connection *Handbook* by William G. Crook, M.D., Square One Publishers, Inc. ©2006. Used by permission of the publisher.

CHAPTER 9

PARASITES

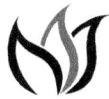

Many do not want to believe they have a parasite issue (the thought is enough to gross-out anyone). Initially it made me feel dirty, but this is not the case as I came to find out. Everyone needs a healthy balance of parasites. The way I look at parasites; they are bottom feeders in an aquarium. Their needed to clean up the tank . They will eat everything including all the crud. Your tank will be cleaner. Plus it adds more oxygen to the tank. They are your helpers; they are not going to hurt any other fish or ourselves.

 Many parasites that host us are acceptable to our body. For example, we have a parasite that lives near ones eyelashes, they assist in keeping the tissues clean. If we have a healthy, functioning digestive system, we are harboring millions of beneficial bacteria in the small intestine. They help us achieve in building B vitamins (which many lack), killing harmful bacteria and other destructive parasites.

Sometimes we can have an overgrowth of parasites that can be detrimental to our health. These parasites feed off your body's nutrients, leaving you starving for nutrients and more prone to attract disease, such as round worms, flatworms (flukes), tapeworms, and pinworms. The sizes varies they can be microscopic to stretching to 30 feet in length. Hookworm (all in the name) will hook itself to the intestinal walls and live off the host's blood. They also leave behind toxins and cause more labor for the organs to keep your blood and body free from further toxicity.

When following any parasite protocol the first that usually comes out is, ascari. It looks like rice and around the same size. Parasites and the overgrowth of yeast (Candida) a destructive organism seem to go hand-in-hand. The yeast gets out of control, and so do parasites. Just as the hulking creature that came out of me, on the 37 day fast.

Example: Like your trash can, parasites want to live in polluted areas. When keeping the body's immune system in poor condition, the parasite thrives and reproduces itself in your most unhealthy organs.

When taking an antibiotic, some of the beneficial bacteria gets destroyed giving harmful parasites the upper hand advantage. If taking an antibiotic, then make sure to replace the beneficial bacteria in your small intestines before the parasites and yeast takes over. EnzymePower (Ch. 10) and live juicing will benefit your body with helpful enzymes or ask your health care professional.

Possible Signs And Symptoms Of Internal Parasites

- Feel tired most of the time
- Have digestive problems (gas, bloating, constipation or diarrhea that come and go but never really clear up)
- Have gastrointestinal symptoms and bulky stools with excess fat in feces
- Suffer with food sensitivities and environmental intolerance
- Developed allergic-like reactions and can't understand why
- Have joint and muscle pains and inflammation often assumed to be arthritis
- Suffer with anemia or iron deficiency (anemia)
- Have hives, rashes, weeping eczema, cutaneous ulcers, swelling, sores, papular lesions, itchy dermatitis
- Suffer with restlessness and anxiety
- Experience multiple awakenings during the night particularly between 2 and 3 am

- Grind your teeth

- Have an excessive amount of bacterial or viral infections

- Depressed

- Difficulty gaining or losing weight no matter what you do

- Did a Candida program which either didn't help at all or helped some-what but you still can't stay away from bread, alcohol, fruit, or fruit juices

- Can't figure out why you don't feel really great and neither can your doctor

- Itchy ears, nose, anus

- Forgetfulness, slow reflexes, gas and bloating, unclear thinking

- Loss of appetite, yellowish face

- Fast heartbeat, heart pain, pain in the navel

- Eating more than normal but still feeling hungry

- Pain in the back, thighs, shoulders

- Lethargy

- Numb hands

- Burning sensation in the stomach

- Drooling while sleeping

- Damp lips at night, dry lips during the day, grinding teeth while asleep

- Bed wetting

- Women: problems with the menstrual cycle

- Men: sexual dysfunction

Herbal Solution

The three herbs that are very effective in killing parasites are:

- Black walnut

- Wormwood

- Cloves

Also, munch on raw pumpkin seeds. If baking the seeds it will start killing off or decreasing the benefits received from them, again EAT RAW.

If only taking one herbal formula that is working on one phase of the parasites life, that formula will not work on the next phases they will re-hatch and grow again. The procedure that is the chosen one to follow does not happen overnight but does not take forever, either.

These herbs can be found at health food stores along with other herbal combinations. I tried several herbal combinations and felt more success with Dr. Clark's parasite protocol at www.curezone.com. Her company also sells the herbal formulas that she recommends at www.drclarkstore. com. Also, check out how to make your own products mentioned in Chapter 19.

CHAPTER 10

ARE YOU LACKING ENZYMES?

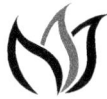

Do you encounter some of these ailments?

- heartburn
- gas
- constipation
- bloating
- lack of energy
- weight issues

These identify the most typical symptoms that been associated to the lack of enzymes, which can create a reduced functioning of the immune system. Beneficial digestive enzymes can be useful for more things than most people realize.

Importance of Digestive Enzymes

The physical body cannot absorb nutrients in food unless there is a sufficient amount of digestive enzymes to break them down. The body progressively loses its ability to produce enzymes on its own. Your body will experience a substantial reduction; roughly every 10 years. In the beginning, it may not be noticeable. Later on, one may discover that their not enjoying nor tolerating certain foods as previously. What this all means is that one is running short of enzymes.

When your body is searching for the missing enzymes, there is considerable stress upon your body. Leaving one with less energy for the other body parts to, function properly.

Enzymes Facts

In addition to fats, carbohydrates, and water, there are enzymes that are required for proper, metabolic function. There are at least 13 kinds of vitamins and 20 kinds of minerals, which are essential nutrients the body needs to, carry out normal bodily functions. They cannot be created on their own they must come from an external source to support the body rebuild. When consuming food it gets broken down, absorbed, and assimilated throughout your body. Nutrients and enzymes act as catalysts, for these processes.

How Enzymes Work

Enzymes being secreted throughout the gastro-intestinal tract and they control the ability to break down food properly. Digestive enzymes are in full force from fresh live raw foods. When foods are cooked, the enzymes, along with vitamins and minerals, are destroyed. Live juicing is the natural way to ensure that one is getting a multitude of enzymes.

Don't worry! You will not keel over from too many.

The true beauty is when live whole foods are in their natural state; you will assume and assimilate the vitamins, minerals and nutrients of what you need and your body will expel what you do not need.

My Enzyme Supplement: EnzymePower

This recipe has hundreds of enzymes, rather than taking a pill that only has a few enzymes. For many, this has given instant freedom from heartburn, bloating, belching after eating, and a stomach that keeps one up all night when the food is not processing sufficiently. Read about EnzymePower in Appendix A.

CHAPTER 11

FOOD TALK

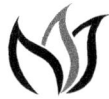

Wheatgrass Benefits

The benefits of Wheatgrass are outstanding. Never knock the power of wheatgrass — it will benefit one from head to toe. The biggest nutritional value of wheatgrass is Chlorophyll which makes up over 70% of the solid content of wheatgrass juice. This is the basis of all plant life. Chlorophyll often referred to as "the blood of plant life," and closely resembles the molecules of human, red blood cells. It will benefit one in every way, shape and form. One to two ounces of wheatgrass is equivalent to 10 pounds of vegetables. Imagine sticking 10 pounds of vegetables in a juicing machine and how many ounces one would have to drink.

Wheatgrass is a powerful detoxifier, and it is especially beneficial to your blood and liver. The enzymes and amino acids found in wheatgrass can protect us from many toxic substances like no other food or medicine can.

The juice bar at a local health food store made me my mere, first shot of wheatgrass. When she handed it to me, I looked at it and thought, "Ewe – that is pretty green!" Regardless, down-the-hatch it went, and I was quite surprised to discover how truly sweet wheatgrass taste.

You have to know my thoughts by now, "a little is good, more is better!"

I then became a wheatgrass junkie. I was on a lengthy fast with not a whole lot of debris left floating in me. I thought, "I am going to try this out," and quadrupled dose of wheatgrass and to see what happened. Within several minutes, my stomach starting churning and I could not get home fast enough to go to the bathroom. Believe me, by this time there should not have been much left in me but just when I thought I was totally cleaned out…was I ever wrong!

Literally, wheatgrass is so safe and beneficial, it can go anywhere from your hooter to your tooter, and on your skin too. Drink it, apply it directly to your skin, or use it in an enema, these are just a few examples of how you can use wheatgrass.

An important question I had about wheatgrass, since it contains the word "wheat", does it contain gluten?

Answer is no. The formation of gluten in wheat is when wheatgrass has grown long enough to become a grain.

The other nice attribute to wheatgrass is that it is not only powerful but also very inexpensive. You can grow wheatgrass right in your own home. It will cost you approximately 3 cents a shot, which is a huge money saver considering it is approximately equivalent to 10 pounds of vegetables.

 You do need a special juicer just for wheatgrass. A juicing machine that you use for vegetables spins too fast and will oxidize the wheatgrass, turning it a brownish color and causing it to lose its sweetness.

For more information about wheatgrass, go to www.annwigmore.com.

Garlic Benefits

Don't forget about garlic and the incredible benefits it has for you. Garlic has a great flavor for cooking and your body will love the benefits it gets from garlic. Garlic contains a substance called Allicin, which has anti-bacterial properties that are equivalent to weak penicillin.

Sure, many have heard of the importance of garlic. Mainly I hear from others that they use it for their blood and they take garlic capsules. Not all herbal supplements are created equally. Just because garlic capsules are in a health food store, does not necessarily mean they are good quality. Fresh is always best. Garlic is an herb that is readily available to you, right now and fresh.

Easy way to remember garlic is an anti, anti everything: Antibiotic, Antifungal, Anticancer, Antibacterial, Antiseptic and I can keep going but I would like to keep your attention. In addition to keeping your heart and blood vessels in a healthy condition, research has proven that garlic lowers your blood pressure, cholesterol, fends off respiratory infections, infections of the urinary tract, and digestive tract. It is reported that garlic is more effective against pathogenic yeasts than Nystatin, especially Candida Albicans.

How to Use Garlic

First buy raw garlic, and not in a jar, either. Once you go fresh you will never go back.

- Consume it with your live juice. When doing so, put it in first before the blade and strainer get filled with other vegetables. That way you will get more of the ANTI benefits from garlic.

- Eat it raw. Take the skin off the clove, put in back of your mouth by the back molars and chomp, which is a must to kick off the medicinal properties that garlic contains the substance called Allicin, which has antibacterial properties that are equivalent to weak penicillin; otherwise you will just poop it out whole with no benefits at all. Immediately wash down with water.

- Apply a sliced clove of garlic directly to your skin, then apply a band-aid or bandage over the garlic to hold it in place.

* NOTE: Garlic will burn and blister the skin. When applying to the skin always rub olive oil in first to act as barrier.

Smell

Worried about the smell of garlic on your breath or seeping through your pores? Simply follow it with peppermint tea, which counteracts the fragrance of garlic. The healthier and more cleansed out one gets, the less smell there is. The stronger odor is a result of it being absorbed into a constipated body.

My Son's Garlic Story

My son, at the age of 8, had a very nasty cold with a fever. Nothing we had helped him get better. He had a big camping trip planned and really, *really* wanted to go on it, in that "the-world-is-going-to-end-if-I-don't-get-to-go" way unique to 8-year-old boys. He wanted to get better, and FAST.

Out of desperation, he was willing to try anything, even my "funky" ideas. He took a shot of Cayenne to help ward off the cold but that was not enough. It was not breaking the fever. He still needed to pump it up a notch. Then we tried garlic. Making it kid friendly way, I minced the garlic and put it in an empty capsule. Right in front of my eyes: GREAT SUCCESS!

The red flushness immediately went away along with the fever. We repeated that evening. My thoughts always go to, "A little is good, more is better."

We repeated this in the morning. We learned because he had an empty stomach, and the garlic being raw in the capsule, the digestive enzymes did not know it was coming down and it cramped his stomach. The moral: when you try this have something in your stomach, whether it is live juice or food.

Healing With Garlic Paste

Are you worried that your child is too young? Or, perhaps you can't stand garlic, even as an adult. SOLUTION: Garlic Paste

This is best applied before bed. It will have time to absorb through your body all night, undisturbed. Mix together:

- 3-10 cloves of garlic minced (according to the size of your feet)
- 1 to 2 tablespoon of Vaseline

Spread this on the bottom of your feet. To hold in place, apply gauze over the garlic paste, then put on socks.

Sugar

We all know how we feel after eating too much sugar versus eating too much broccoli. The broccoli doesn't have the same adverse effect on the body. It will not make us bloated and tired, the way that eating too many candy bars can.

I will tell you what I think the world needs: a Sugar Anonymous group, world-wide. I can see myself in a room, raising my hand, saying, "I am a Sugaraholic!"

Sugar was my main form of food from childhood into adulthood. I would eat enough other food just to earn that dessert. I would rather have lived on candy bars than anything else. I believe the main reason for my various health issues was the over-consumption of sugar.

Sugar will coat the inside of your body and stick there, preventing your body from working properly. My colon was a prime example, with sugar coating the walls of my small to large intestines. Remember my story of the 37-day fast, and the 14 feet of old, dried-up sludgy, grunge that came out of me? I can guarantee that was the product of many candy bars, bottles of pop, cookies etc. Sugar to me is the most addictive substance, and to give that up is TOUGH, real TOUGH. I will say it again – "TOUGH!!"

In addition to throwing off the body's balance, excess sugar (especially processed, white sugar) may result in a large number of other physical ailments. The following list of ailments associated with too much sugar was compiled from a variety of scientific publications.

93 Reasons To Think About What Sugar Can Do

1. SUGAR CAN CAUSE a suppressed immune system
2. SUGAR CAN CAUSE an upset of mineral relationships in the body
3. SUGAR CAN CAUSE hyperactivity
4. SUGAR CAN CAUSE anxiety
5. SUGAR CAN CAUSE difficulty in concentration
6. SUGAR CAN CAUSE crankiness
7. SUGAR CAN CAUSE drowsiness
8. SUGAR CAN CAUSE decreased activity
9. SUGAR CAN CAUSE an adverse affect on children's school grades
10. SUGAR CAN CAUSE a significant rise in triglycerides
11. SUGAR CAN CAUSE impaired defense against bacterial infection (infectious diseases)
12. SUGAR CAN CAUSE loss of tissue elasticity, leading to wrinkles
13. SUGAR CAN CAUSE chromium deficiency

14. SUGAR CAN CAUSE increased fasting levels of glucose
15. SUGAR CAN CAUSE copper deficiency
16. SUGAR CAN CAUSE impaired absorption of calcium and magnesium
17. SUGAR CAN CAUSE weakened eyesight
18. SUGAR CAN CAUSE hypoglycemia
19. SUGAR CAN CAUSE an acidic digestive track
20. SUGAR CAN CAUSE rapid rise in adrenaline levels in children
21. SUGAR CAN CAUSE premature aging
22. SUGAR CAN CAUSE tooth decay
23. SUGAR CAN CAUSE obesity
24. SUGAR CAN CAUSE Chrohns
25. SUGAR CAN CAUSE Ulcerative colitis
26. SUGAR CAN CAUSE arthritis
27. SUGAR CAN CAUSE asthma
28. SUGAR CAN CAUSE Candida Albicians
29. SUGAR CAN CAUSE gallstones
30. SUGAR CAN CAUSE kidney stones
31. SUGAR CAN CAUSE multiple sclerosis
32. SUGAR CAN CAUSE epilepsy
33. SUGAR CAN CAUSE appendicitis
34. SUGAR CAN CAUSE hemorrhoids
35. SUGAR CAN CAUSE varicose veins
36. SUGAR CAN CAUSE periodontal disease
37. SUGAR CAN CAUSE osteoporosis
38. SUGAR CAN CAUSE saliva acidity
39. SUGAR CAN CAUSE decreased insulin sensitivity
40. SUGAR CAN CAUSE cancer
41. SUGAR CAN CAUSE increased cholesterol
42. SUGAR CAN CAUSE increased blood pressure
43. SUGAR CAN CAUSE decreased growth hormones
44. SUGAR CAN CAUSE mal-absorption of protein
45. SUGAR CAN CAUSE food allergies
46. SUGAR CAN CAUSE diabetes
47. SUGAR CAN CAUSE toxemia during pregnancy
48. SUGAR CAN CAUSE eczema in children
49. SUGAR CAN CAUSE cardiovascular disease
50. SUGAR CAN CAUSE the creation of collagen
51. SUGAR CAN CAUSE cataracts

52. SUGAR CAN CAUSE emphysema
53. SUGAR CAN CAUSE arthrosclerosis
54. SUGAR CAN CAUSE a lowering of enzymes' ability to function
55. SUGAR CAN CAUSE Parkinson's
56. SUGAR CAN CAUSE an increase in the body's fluid retention
57. SUGAR CAN CAUSE constipation
58. SUGAR CAN CAUSE nearsightedness
59. SUGAR CAN CAUSE tendons to be more brittle
60. SUGAR CAN CAUSE headaches
61. SUGAR CAN CAUSE migraines
62. SUGAR CAN CAUSE learning disorders
63. SUGAR CAN CAUSE depression
64. SUGAR CAN CAUSE Alzheimer's
65. SUGAR CAN CAUSE hormonal imbalance
66. SUGAR CAN CAUSE dizziness
67. SUGAR CAN CAUSE feeding of cancer cells
68. SUGAR CAN CAUSE addiction
69. SUGAR CAN CAUSE intoxication, like alcohol
70. SUGAR CAN CAUSE exacerbated PMS
71. SUGAR CAN CAUSE chronic degenerative diseases
72. SUGAR CAN CAUSE epileptic seizures
73. SUGAR CAN CAUSE an induced cell death
74. SUGAR CAN CAUSE mild memory loss
75. SUGAR CAN CAUSE IBS
76. SUGAR CAN CAUSE brain decay
77. SUGAR CAN CAUSE metabolic syndrome
78. SUGAR CAN CAUSE gray hair
79. SUGAR CAN CAUSE ulcers
80. SUGAR CAN CAUSE gout
81. SUGAR CAN CAUSE premature aging
82. SUGAR CAN CAUSE an increase in the amount of liver fat
83. SUGAR CAN CAUSE a slowdown of adrenal gland function
84. SUGAR CAN CAUSE the risk of Polio
85. SUGAR CAN CAUSE ADHD
86. SUGAR CAN CAUSE an adverse effect to the nervous system
87. SUGAR CAN CAUSE schizophrenia
88. SUGAR CAN CAUSE slowing of food in the gastrointestinal tract
89. SUGAR CAN CAUSE mucous in your body

90. SUGAR CAN CAUSE an increased size of the liver by dividing the liver cells
91. SUGAR CAN CAUSE compromised lining of the capillaries
92. SUGAR CAN CAUSE platelet adhesiveness
93. SUGAR CAN CAUSE emotional instability

Now, have I gotten you to think what sugar does? In a nutshell, it coats, sticks, and plasters to the inside of your body, to every living organ and cell, preventing them from working properly. This all falls under the old adage, "you are what you eat."

The good news, it is never too late to clean it up by following one of the programs that I have listed: Mucous-Diet Free diet, JuicePower Fasting, or PowerHouse Healing Fast. Once you follow these protocols, you will feel better and ailments will start subsiding. It is all in the choices we make. Let's all become the VICTOR by simply controlling what goes in.

Cayenne: The King of Herbs

Cayenne means any hot pepper. I find it necessary to let you know about the extreme benefits of cayenne. If you are ever in doubt, just try it!

1. CAYENNE CAN HELP abscesses
2. CAYENNE CAN HELP acne
3. CAYENNE CAN HELP allergies
4. CAYENNE CAN HELP arthritis
5. CAYENNE CAN HELP asthma & respiratory conditions
6. CAYENNE CAN HELP aura brilliance
7. CAYENNE CAN HELP bladder infection
8. CAYENNE CAN HELP bleeding internal and externally
9. CAYENNE CAN HELP blood pressure
10. CAYENNE CAN HELP blood sugar levels
11. CAYENNE CAN HELP bronchitis
12. CAYENNE CAN HELP bruises
13. CAYENNE CAN HELP bursitis
14. CAYENNE CAN HELP burns
15. CAYENNE CAN HELP cardiovascular disease
16. CAYENNE CAN HELP cholesterol and triglyceride levels
17. CAYENNE CAN HELP circulatory system

18. CAYENNE CAN HELP common cold
19. CAYENNE CAN HELP cramps
20. CAYENNE CAN HELP digestive system
21. CAYENNE CAN HELP drowning victim
22. CAYENNE CAN HELP dyspepsia
23. CAYENNE CAN HELP fatigue
24. CAYENNE CAN HELP fever
25. CAYENNE CAN HELP flatulence
26. CAYENNE CAN HELP flu
27. CAYENNE CAN HELP frostbite
28. CAYENNE CAN HELP fungal infection
29. CAYENNE CAN HELP hangover
30. CAYENNE CAN HELP headache
31. CAYENNE CAN HELP heart attack
32. CAYENNE CAN HELP heat exhaustion
33. CAYENNE CAN HELP herpes
34. CAYENNE CAN HELP high blood pressure
35. CAYENNE CAN HELP hypothermia
36. CAYENNE CAN HELP increase energy levels
37. CAYENNE CAN HELP increase libido
38. CAYENNE CAN HELP indigestion
39. CAYENNE CAN HELP induce perspiration, which actually helps a person
40. CAYENNE CAN HELP to cool off and releases toxins
41. CAYENNE CAN HELP inflammation
42. CAYENNE CAN HELP intestinal inflammation
43. CAYENNE CAN HELP kidney problems
44. CAYENNE CAN HELP low back pain
45. CAYENNE CAN HELP low blood pressure
46. CAYENNE CAN HELP memory
47. CAYENNE CAN HELP menstrual cramps
48. CAYENNE CAN HELP migraine
49. CAYENNE CAN HELP nose bleeds CAYENNE CAN HELP
50. CAYENNE CAN HELP peripheral neuropathy
51. CAYENNE CAN HELP post-surgical pain
52. CAYENNE CAN HELP post herpetic neuralgia
53. CAYENNE CAN HELP prevent blood clots
54. CAYENNE CAN HELP psoriasis & other skin conditions
55. CAYENNE CAN HELP pyorrhea of the gums

56. CAYENNE CAN HELP scalds
57. CAYENNE CAN HELP shingles
58. CAYENNE CAN HELP shock
59. CAYENNE CAN HELP simple back strains
60. CAYENNE CAN HELP skin cancer
61. CAYENNE CAN HELP sore muscles
62. CAYENNE CAN HELP sprains
63. CAYENNE CAN HELP stroke
64. CAYENNE CAN HELP sunburns
65. CAYENNE CAN HELP tonsillitis
66. CAYENNE CAN HELP toothache
67. CAYENNE CAN HELP ulcers
68. CAYENNE CAN HELP unclear thinking
69. CAYENNE CAN HELP urinary tract infection
70. CAYENNE CAN HELP varicella viruses
71. CAYENNE CAN HELP varicose veins
72. CAYENNE CAN HELP vision &night blindness
73. CAYENNE CAN HELP weight loss

When in doubt, just give it a try!

CLEANSING AND FASTING PROTOCOLS

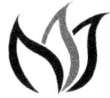

CHAPTER 12

FASTING GUIDELINES

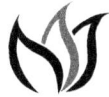

Once you establish your mindset, fasting really is quite simple. Making and keeping yourself healthy is at your fingertips and not out of reach. It is a really great feeling to have that much control over your own health.

Missing Component

You name it, I tried it! Many times there is a missing component of putting all the pieces of the pie together for natural healing.

One of the missing components to natural healing is giving the body a break to fix itself, and that is accomplished by fasting. Healing does not have to take years, or even months.

With just fasting alone, it did not work any significant length of time. I always ended up returning to fasting.

If you are asking yourself," Why, did she keep returning?"

It worked, immediately on the symptoms that I was experiencing. It would stop the pain of Optic Neuritis dead in its tracks from the very first day of a fast.

Following the pain was deteriorating vision, and being on a fast it would stop at the pain and not go any further. When I lost control of my fingers, and could not open a car door, nor button my jeans. Every day on a fast I had seen great improvement, from the previous day.

Fasting was always a short term fix. Until I figured out, the missing component to healing my body. A very simplified method, gives your body a break with these, 3 simple steps.

1. Cleanse
2. Nourish
3. Let Thy Body Heal Itself

What Should I Do Before Fasting?

These 3 painless pointers will prepare you for an easier journey into fasting:

- Mucous-Free Diet prior to the fast, your body will be more receptive to lighter amounts of food and will prepare your taste buds for healthy produce.
- Get you colon moving by taking an herbal supplement such as PowerPoop for 2 to 4 weeks, this is a must so you can move into the PowerGrab formula right away.
- Drink plenty of water (preferably distilled).

How Long Should I Fast?

Longer fasting gives the body uninterrupted time to do the work of healing. The 30-day juice fast is a standard in European health facilities. Less than 30 days and you can be missing the best, and rare experiences of the fast.

It takes 60% of your energy to break down solid food. When your body does not have to use its energy to break down food the existing energy will go where the healing needs to be.

I have found with all the fasting that I did, that the longer ones were much more effective as opposed to the shorter ones. As evidence, most of the recoveries from my illnesses have taken place in the latter parts of longer fasting periods, with live juice in combination with water only.

This is where your choices come in and what you want to accomplish. You can start, slow or go gun-ho. This when you have to ask yourself, "What do I want to accomplish, little healing or a lot?"

- One day
- Several days
- Week
- 10 days
- 14 days
- 30 days
- Seasonally
- Once a year

To see more lasting changes, it is highly recommended too fast:

- 14 to 30 days

 The body will direct you to what you need and the appropriate length of time for you. If you recall from my story, I trusted my body. When I knew the live juice was not giving me results that I needed, that is when I started the water fast. I knew it was right with all the healing I was receiving daily and the energy level kept rising. I continued it until my energy began to drop, and then I resumed the live juice and my energy levels went back up again. Just listen to your body.

The 1-Day Fast

Another fasting idea is a one-day fast. Drink different types of juice, but take no food or other liquid.

Most of us have never gone without food for longer than a few hours. Begin with short fasts, and gradually move for longer periods of time if you desire. Be prepared for some dizziness, headache, or nausea in the early stages, and those symptoms may or may never happen. These symptoms may also come from constipation in your colon. You will notice some symptoms leave after you had a decent bowel movement.

Not too long ago, I did a small fast for 3 days and I was doing everything correctly. I had a nagging pain in my head, which was unusual as I am not prone to head-aches. The following morning I still had the nagging pain in my head until, I had a decent bowel movement and the pain in my head flushed away with everything else. Headache pains can be caused from your feces stuck in the weak area of the transverse part of your colon. Massaging counter clockwise the transverse area of your colon. Massaging will assist in the release of feces and move it out faster.

As you do more of this fasting you will become more in tune with what you body is doing and why. At that time, you will understand the simplicity and importance of regular fasting.

Water Only

The 10-day water fast has also become a recommended number of days. Paul Bragg is an advocate of the 10-day water fast. In most cases 10 days on water will cause the same weight loss as 30 days on juice. But water-fasting is far more difficult, especially if you have a fast metabolism. The trick to any fasting is the *PowerGrab* formula. It will bulk up in your digestive system causing a feeling of fullness, plus nutritious.

The turning point of where the, "feeling of the healing," eventually came to me on the 37 day fast, it was with water/salt and herbal formulas only, from Day Six to Day Sixteen.

Alternating

Alternating between juice and water fasting is the most effective method of achieving a full cleansing. The juice fasting is used when you need the energy to work or get things done. When you are alternating between juice and water, the juice will give your body liquid nutrition that you will assume, assimilate, and store for the water fasting. You should always include two of three days of juice fasting before and after the water fast.

Consult with your physician to be sure you are medically able to fast before attempting it.

Think Salt

For all fasts, especially water only fasting, think salt.

A good sea salt is best and highest in mineral content. Use a measuring teaspoon. The rule of thumb is 1/8 teaspoon for every 16 oz.; 1/4 teaspoon for every 32 oz

(I quart); 1/2 teaspoon for 64 oz., or I full teaspoon for I gallon. (Some people will need less salt, others more). This is a starting point, not a set rule. You can just add the salt to your juice or add the salt to the water and shake or stir it. The best way is to just throw the salt into your mouth and chase it with water.

If you recall my 37 day fast, the benefit of sea salt was amazing; it resulted in the death of that creature inside my colon, which was then finally expelled. I would not recommend someone to do what I did at that moment, it was too excessive. Although, there were no side effects accept the surprise from the sight of the creature that came out of me.

NOTE: If your ankles, fingers, or eyelids swell, don't do the salt for two days, just drink the water. Then on the 3rd day begin taking the salt again. If your kidneys are not working well, then don't follow this program. If you still want to try it on your own, just drink one eight-ounce glass of water and wait until you go to the bathroom. Then drink another glass. When your kidneys come up to speed (input matches output), then start the salt slowly to make sure your kidneys are working ok. Always consult with your health care provider.

Breaking a Fast

After a prolonged fast, be easy on your digestive system.

- Eat slow and light
- Wholesome Mucous-Free foods
- Keep on juicing
- Plenty of water

The difficulty with any length of a fasting is to not overeat after you're done. You may be tempted to reward yourself for being so diligent.

Don't give in now! When you fall into temptation and eat the wrong foods, the benefits you just gained will evaporate quickly. Even overeating fruit can cause problems. Always remember: treat fruit as a desert and keep in mind moderation.

Common Fasting Questions

Q: I don't like vegetables; can I fast only on fruit juice?

A: Yes, JuicePower Fast.

Q: Can I have coffee when I fast?

A: No caffeine. Herbal teas are a great alternative.

Q: Should I stop all supplements?

A: Your choice and you may find what Hippocrates said, "Let food be thy medicine, medicine will be thy food." You may come to a point of realization, how powerful food is and when you are getting blasted with nutrients from live juicing.

Q: Should I fast while I have an ill-working colon or should I fix that first?

A: If you have time prior to a fast, it is ideal to get it moving first. You will also find the fasting itself will assist in repairing an ill-working colon.

Q: Should I do less while fasting?

A: That depends on you and your energy level. It never stopped me from doing extra activity.

Q: Is the first fast the hardest?

A: Depends on you. Get yourself prepared mentally for what you want to accomplish. Some have to put themselves in a position that will not be tempting to them to cave in. Do whatever you have to do and once you do, it is not a big deal.

Q: How long before I start feeling benefits?

A: Depends on your body and how much effort you put into these protocols. Generally, clients of mine will experience some improvement in the first 24 hours, and then experience bigger changes the longer they maintain the fast. Personally, I have felt relief as early as the first day, but there was one time when it was not until the 6th day.

Q: How long does it take for the hunger to go away?

A: When you feel hunger pains, you can curb that with drinking more water or live juice. There is no maximum limit to the quantity of liquids that you consume. Plus, if you add the *PowerGrab* capsules, you will be consuming up to 50 capsules a day, it will bulk up in your digestive system and provide you the sense of fullness which makes the endeavor much easier.

Q: How do you wash all these fruits and vegetable?

A: Fill the sink with water and add two tablespoons of apple cider vinegar in the water. Let it soak for about 5 minutes, rinse and drain. You want a superior quality of apple cider vinegar that has the floaters at the bottom, called the mother of apple cider vinegar. I prefer the Braggs brand.

Q: How much weight do you lose when you fast?

A: First day is consistently the most significant drop from excess fluid retention. It all depends on your body weight and if you have excess to lose. After the first day, the loss is 1 pound a day till I have reached my ideal body weight, then it comes to a screeching halt.

Q: Will I lose too much weight?

A: Getting your organs cleansed out will have an impact to balancing your body's weight. Fasting may allow you to gain additional weight before or afterwards.

Example: on my 37 day fast I had a good 25 pounds to lose. When my weight was at 130 pounds, I felt great. I did not lose another pound even though I continued for seven more days. Your body will know what to do and where to stop. It is smart!

Q: How can one go without food, fiber, and nutrition?

A: The produce you will be consuming has a countless amount of nutrition, protein and calories. In fact, with live juicing, your body will be blasted with nutrients, far more than you get in an average day. Your body safely can go without solid food up to 30 days but never without water.

Q: Will I gain all my weight back after the fast?

A: Answer is simple. It is up to you.

More great news!

You now have lost more than just inches of fat. Fasting changes your filters inside you. You need to reintroduce a clean, lean, youthful body to a healthful diet. It would not be in your best interest to reward yourself with the lazy, junk-food lifestyle you once lived. If doing so, the answer will be yes, the weight and other ailments that you suffered from will gladly come home. You have exercised authority over food. Reward yourself with healthy foods for your accomplishment, that some may have never thought was possible.

Q: Can I exercise while fasting?

A: Absolutely you need to do so. It will oxygenate your blood and promotes circulation, which helps with healing at a faster pace. Energy during a fast can be fickle. Some will encounter an abundance of energy making exercise easy and fun. If you experience an energy loss, limit yourself to stretching exercises, light walking, or deep breathing.

Q: How much should I drink?

A: There is no upper nor lower limit to the amount of live juice one should consume.

Q: Should I continue with my medication?

A: Some do successfully fast while on medication. Some will find they never need to turn back to taking their medication, with the healing they experience. Supernatural things happen when fasting.

If you must take medication and intend to fast then I recommend you do the juice fast. The vegetable juices will help protect the stomach from harsh pharmaceutical medications. I wouldn't recommend taking pharmaceutical medications when you are doing water only. Always consult your doctor regarding the effect of fasting combined with your medication.

Q: If I smoke, do I need to quit while fasting?

A: The perfect world, yes. If you need to smoke while fasting, you may find the longer you go on a fast, you will lose the desire and urge. Getting your body cleansed out, and blasted with nutrients will make your efforts of quitting, if you desire, much easier.

If you desire to quit, this leads me to a potential solution for you. There is a wonderful book called *Easy Way To Quit Smoking* by Allen Carr. Get that book and read it. He suggests logical thoughts that makes quitting smoking easier. I know — been there, done that. The more your body gets cleansed out, and you build your nutrition, you will find it this makes it easier for you to reach your goal of quitting smoking.

I recommend LobeliaPower Tincture. It helps calm you down, plus it makes cigarettes taste terrible. The Indians used to call it their wacky ta Baky, because of the calming effect.

Q: Can I do a fast if I have diabetes?

With there being a couple of different types of Diabetic condition, it will entirely depend on the type. You can always do a Mucous-Free diet and juicing, while cleansing out your organs.

You can control the types of sugar that one may need, more greens for a lower carb count, or one that needs more sugar, use the higher carb count of fruits and vegetables while eating or drinking.

Always consult your physician first.

Q: Can I do this if I am underweight?

When someone is under or overweight there is an unbalance in your body that is creating this to happen. It can be an overgrowth of Candida or parasites in either case.

For someone underweight, your body knows what to do and take care of itself. You may loss a couple but do not be surprised if you stay close to the same weight or put on weight during the fasting protocol. Just as I was on that fast for 37 days, why did I not I lose any more weight on the last 7 days? There was nothing different. My body finished losing weight, and it knew what to do.

Slippery Elm is the beneficial herb, to assist in gaining weight. Slippery Elm Gruel (slimy consistency) the name explains it. Take one tablespoon (adult size) mix with a cup of hot water, stir well and if too slimy for you, decrease the amount. Looks bad, but does not taste bad. Do this 3 times a day. *PowerGrab* has Slippery Elm already in the formula.

Q: Will fasting shrink my stomach?

A: Fasting helps recover the stomach's natural elasticity, restoring a flat stomach. You will remain satisfied on less food, in proportionate size to the body's caloric requirements. If you would like to obtain a flatter stomach, you can safely exercise the abdominal muscles every day even on a fast.

Q: Since I have finished fasting, why am I more sensitive to unhealthy food?

A: Now don't be complaining about this one. After a fast your body is clean and has far less tolerance to the toxic foods that you were eating previous to the fast. You will be much more aware of your body after this point. Feeling ill from eating junk-food is a sign that your body is, functioning normally.

Fasting restores the body's potential for violently reacting to harmful, health-damaging food. Oh sure, you can desensitize your body by slowly introducing harmful foods into your diet. And before you know it all the good performed by the fast will be undone. Perish the thought! Having a healthy body may restrict your ability to tolerate what you were previously open to indulge in.

Q: Should I abstain from sexual relations during a fast?

A: No, in fact you may have an increased libido on a fast and the sex might be better than before.

Personal Note: I used to have a discomfort of pressure during intercourse and since the fasting all of that pain vanished.

Q: Can you fast when you have a chronic or terminal illness?

A: The only time it will hurt you is when you do nothing. Some may have to dive into it slower than others depending on the toxicity of their body, and toxins may start being eliminated too fast for fragile bodies. If fasting is not going to work or if you need a starting point, the Mucous-Free diet is another excellent option. It just takes longer to reach the finish line, but heading towards that line.

Always remember, it is better to do something rather than nothing at all.

Q: Am I going to be tired all the time?

A: Good news: there are more up days then down days. The up days you will have so much energy and get so much more done then you do in a typical day. Then on the down days, you may need to rest or take it easy. Do not worry, it will pass shortly. The most pertinent part is to make sure you are getting enough nutrition. That makes a world of a difference. When I embarked on the water fasting I had 6 days prior of live juicing.

Add-In To All The Protocols

Water

Water itself is a wonder healer for your body; I have seen so many tremendous benefits with just simply drinking water. I have even fasted with water alone for 10 days.

I prefer DISTILLED water.

The reason for this is that distilled water is 'thirsty' water. It will help grab the inorganic minerals and salts in your body.

Your body is made up of 80% fluids, so you need to replenish it daily with water. When focusing on cleansing out your body, drink a gallon each day. If you want a more technical way to determine the amount, take your body weight and divide it by 2 — that number is how many ounces you should drink per day. For example, if you weigh 125 pounds, then you should drink 63 ounces of water a day. A great book to read about water is *Your Body's Many Cries For Water*, by Fereydoon Batmanghelidj.

Are you still asking yourself, "Why distilled water?"

Here is a testimonial on why:

Dear Gina,

Just wanted to tell you how well your recommendation to drink distilled water worked!!!! I had gone in for my annual exam, and the doctor said there were traces of blood and crystals in my urine, indicating the start of kidney stones. Over the next two or three weeks, I was checked two more times, with the same result, and so I was sent to an urologist. I started drinking distilled water and, by the time I got to the urologist, he couldn't figure out why I was there! There were no traces of blood or crystals. He even had to double check the test results that were sent to his office. He wanted to know what I had been doing, because it was obviously working — and he couldn't believe it was something so simple!

– Julie from Chicago

Distilled water will grab the inorganic salts and mineral. Remember when your mom used to put distilled water in the iron? Her motivation for doing so was to avoid a mineral deposit build-up, so it would not clog up the iron.

Your body is like that good ole' pressing iron used by your grandma and mom. They did not want minerals to clog up their iron; why would you want your body to be clogged up? You might be thinking that this only applies to your kidneys, but no, it is from head to toe (Including your joints, organs, and blood.)

Hydrotherapy

There is much power in this treatment; do not sell this short. Alternate hot and cold water in your shower; if you have access to a sauna, then it will be extremely beneficial, as well. Do this daily to promote more circulation. Place your whole body, in a very HOT shower, for a minute; then turn it all the way to cold. YES! All the way to cold, then go back to hot, then cold, then hot, etc. Aim for 7 minutes, going back and forth with the hot/cold. You can aim the water on certain parts of your body.

You will feel revitalized after this and have a ton of energy. In addition, it is a great for promoting deep breathing. Remember, circulation is crucial for healing the body. When a part of your body is ill or hurting; there is a lack of circulation to that area.

High Enema And Colonics

It should not be used as a crutch; it is only a helper for getting your body detoxified. It takes time to eliminate a lifetime of debris of stuck waste! An enema in a disposable bottle (approx. 6 ounces), works on the lower bowel. High enemas go much further. Enemas can be used daily or weekly when cleansing, and detoxifying.

Colonic

If a colonic specialist is within your financial means, then I highly recommend getting one. The sessions consist of about an hour of water going in and out of your colon, and they are well worth it! The cost of colonics can be $60.00 and up, per session. In some areas, you can find schools that offer such sessions at reduced costs. During my PowerHouse Protocol, once a week I received colonics.

High Enema

What you need for a High Enema:
- A enema bag that holds 2 to 4 quarts of water.

- *Optional:* You can use herbal teas in your enema. Use 2-3 tbs. of herb and 1 cup of hot water, steep; add to enema bag with the rest of the water.

Here are some suggestions for the use of herbs mixed in with your 2nd cool enema: cayenne, raspberry leaves, catnip, chickweed, white oak bark, shepherd's purse, echinacea, strawberry leaves, raspberry leaves, wheatgrass, kelp and some use coffee to stimulate the liver. Dissolve 1 or 2 *PowerPoop* capsules, in hot water, steep, strain, and add it to the second cooler enema. Always, strain the herbs, otherwise the herbs will get stuck in the enema tip.

I had a client mix 1 cup of olive oil to her mixture of water to the enema bag to help assist herself for a smoother movement. It was a success and lessened her pain that she was going through to get the blockage removed.

Most healthy adults can easily take 2 quarts of solution with little or no discomfort.

It is better to do something, rather than nothing.

How to Administer a High Enema

1. Place yourself in the most comfortable and convenient area near the toilet as possible; you can do the enema on your bathroom floor, bed etc. If bedridden, get a container or bedpan that it can be expelled into.

2. Lying on your left side, with the right leg flexed, this position enables the enema solution to flow smoothly into the rectum & sigmoid colon.

3. Fill the enema bag with warm water. Warmth will help you to expel faster.

4. The nozzle can be lubricated (Vaseline) for easier insertion and inserted into the rectum about 2 to 6 inches. Inject the water slowly to help reduce discomfort. It is also beneficial to breathe slowly and deeply through the mouth. This will help reduce discomfort in your abdomen and enable you to take the high enema more effectively. If you experience cramps slow down or halt the solution, momentarily.

5. Massage abdomen in a counter-clockwise direction to help advance the solution higher into the colon and assist you to accept more of the enema solution.

6. As the solution is moving through you, shift your body position. From

your starting position of lying on your left side, gently and slowly roll onto your back, then on right side. This will make it natural flow in the direction of your large intestines.

7. Once the enema is administered, you will probably experience the urgency to move the bowels. Relax and hold it for 5 – 10 minutes. If you cannot hold it that long, then that's okay too.

8. Expel the warm water into the toilet. When expelling the enema, massaging the abdomen clockwise helps to move the solution and feces through the rectum and out the anus.

9. Follow it with a second enema of 2 to 4 qts. of cooler water. The cool water will assist the colon to contract and you will be able to hold it in longer. (You may add your herbal preparation to the water if desired). Be easy and gentle. You will experience a sense of fullness, but never pain.

10. During this enema, take in as much of the enema solution as possible to make certain that your entire large intestine is completely filled and distended.

11. Repeat the rolling and massaging pattern as before.

12. Relax and hold for 5 – 15 minutes. Expel the water into the toilet.

13. You may need to obtain a second container for the additional water if the bag is not large enough.

Exercise

Find something you like to do — walking, running, trampoline — just do something! Get your heart going, get some sun, and have some FUN!

Skin Brushing

To help slough off old, dead, and dry skin cells so the skin can breathe. Brush your skin, always going toward your heart. A natural sable brush is a better choice for skin brushing and creating more circulation and sloughing off dead skin cells. You can find sable brushes at your local health food stores. If you do not have one, do not sweat it; use a loofah pad or if all you have is a washcloth then use it. Anything is better than nothing.

Juicer

A juicer is a must have. It will blast your body inside and out with nutrition. The outstanding results one would never receive out of a jar; there is no comparison. With all the nutrients, minerals and enzymes one receives through juicing, you will experience more vitality, energy, and healthier sleep. What more could anyone want?

Many people confuse juice extractors with the blenders that are in their kitchens, but juice extractors are completely different machines. A juice extractor is a device that mechanically separates juice from the solid part (pulp) of most fruits, vegetables, leafy greens, and herbs.

There are three main types of juicers:

- Centrifugal juicers: use blades and a sieve to separate juice from the pulp.
- Masticating juicers: 'chew' fruit to a pulp before squeezing out the juice.
- Triturating juicers: have twin gears to first crush fruit and then press it.

Masticating and triturating juicers can also juice wheatgrass. By contrast, centrifugal juicers cannot break the fibers of the grass, and the centrifugal juicer's speed would oxidize the wheatgrass, turning it brown in color and losing the sweet flavor of the wheatgrass.

You can search online for all different types of juicers. The one that I started with was the Juiceman JR®. It worked, and you can pick up that juicer for about $60.00 at Target, K-Mart, etc. It is more along the lines of a disposable juicer; it does not have a long life-span, but that is okay. It is a terrific starter. (The other place to search, if you have time, is in the second-hand stores.)

I own a Champion Juicer and Omega Juicer. When you get into the more costly ones like those, they are worth it! You use much less produce. I personally think the juice tastes better – and we all know what I think about taste! I like it!!! I prefer a machine that ejects the pulp, rather than a centrifugal one, because it does not become easily unbalanced and want to eject from your countertop.

What you can do with the pulp from the juicer?

It seems like a waste to throw it away. You can save it for recipes of soups or salads, compost, or I feed it to my dog with a mixture of raw meat.

For my dog, I mix and stir well:

- 1/4 pulp from the juicer
- 3/4 raw meats (ground beef, deer, lamb, etc.)
- Warm water so it brings it down to their body temperature, enough to make it into the consistency of a stew
- 1 or 2 tablespoons of *AnimalPower Food*

The Real Secret to Making Flushes Successful

Mindset. Get excited for yourself for this incredible journey you are about to embark on. It is exciting, all the changes your body is going to go through and how much power you have now under your own fingertips. You will directly own your destination by "keeping your eye on the prize."

Smile and have some fun! This will be easy, on the fast one will experience clarity, and it feels as if a cloud has been lifted from your thoughts. Do things that are out of your norm. Get rid of anger, give a gift or other gesture to someone that you had a grievance with, or just drop off a present to someone anonymously. It will boost your spirits and leave you in a different mindset.

Learn something new each day. Learn something new each day. Whether it is a word, a helpful tip, or a joke. It makes one attractive to others and yourself.

Be kind. One can never go wrong with kindness, never needs explaining, and it will enliven your spirit.

Let's Get Ready: A Bit Of Tough Love

I do not want others to suffer needlessly as, I did. I was in way too much pain; if I had not realized there was a way out, I could not have survived and would want to die. It was that bad! What I am saying is, "Stop pussy-footing around!" with all the other stuff. Yes, this takes some dedication and perseverance. It is worth it! Restore your health and grab hold of your own power; welcome your life back through cleansing and fasting.

CHAPTER 13

BASIC – Flushing the Colon, Liver, Kidneys, & Blood

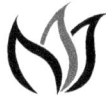

Order of Cleansing Out Your Body

Follow this EASY order. This is where the herbs come in to assist:

1. COLON FLUSH – Get the colon moving for at least 2 to 4 weeks prior to trying any of these protocols. Use a detoxifying and cathartic formula such as *PowerPoop Intestinal Formula*. Once the colon gets moving after 2 to 4 weeks, then you will be ready to move into *PowerGrab* the powerful purifier and intestinal vacuum. It draws the old, hardened fecal matter off the walls of the small intestines and colon and out of any diverticula.

> *Optimum results happen when on a fast. If time permits, always get the colon moving 2 weeks prior to embarking on a fast for better results

2. LIVER FLUSH – The colon must be moving prior to a liver flush as the stones expel through the colon. You must complete at least the 2 week bowel detoxification and **continue** taking the intestinal formula (*PowerPoop*) while completing this program. Then you may either do the 5-day Gentle Liver Flush or the PowerHouse Liver Flush as explained in Chapter 13 . The liver usually is detoxified before the kidneys, but you may reverse this, if desired.

3. KIDNEY FLUSH – Kidneys are generally overworked and often end up heavily infected, inflamed, with crystalline growths, or kidney stones. The herbal products which you will be using on the Kidney Flush are, *CayennePower*, *DetoxPower Tea* and *KidneyPower*. If you are on the PowerHouse fast, omit all sweeteners.

4. BLOOD FLUSH – Finally, your colon, liver and kidneys are done and it is time to move into cleansing the blood. The walls of our veins, arteries, and capillaries become coated with inorganic waste materials, not allowing the cell structures to be fed. This waste forms a lining just as it does in the intestine. If on the 30 day fast, you can start the *PowerBlood Cleansing Tincture* on the last week, even as other cleansings continuing with colon, liver and kidneys.

1st Cleansing - Colon Flush

When the colon is not moving, nothing else is going to continue moving. So get it going! This flush is CRITICAL to complete BEFORE beginning the other flushes and fasts. The more effort that one puts into these protocols, better results you will get. It took years to build-up the gunk and debris currently lining your intestinal walls. This whole cleansing will not materialize overnight. The exciting news: it will not take as long to clean as it took you to get there in the first place.

What You Will Need

- 1st-*PowerPoop Intestinal Formula*
- 2nd-*PowerGrab Intestinal Formula*

PowerPoop Intestinal Formula is a formula designed to get the colon moving which will strengthen and tone your peristaltic muscle. The goal is to get the peristaltic muscle to the point of being useful again and functioning on its own.

PowerGrab Intestinal Formula is a formula designed to grab the heavy metal, toxins, solidify debris stuck to the intestines walls, smothering and grabbing Candida, parasites and assists in healing the intestinal wall.

Weeks 1 &2

You need to stay with the *PowerPoop* for at least 2 weeks minimum before moving into *PowerGrab*. Depending on your system, this may stretch into 3 to 4 weeks. Pay attention to your body and trust what it needs. Once you get that under control (and you will feel it), you will feel much better and different ailments will go away: aches and pains, bloating, constipation, etc.

Week 3

Now you will start *PowerGrab*, which draws out all the old garbage and sludge that is stuck to your gut and intestinal walls (or, as I love to say, from your hooter to your tooter).

Take *PowerGrab* capsules 7 to 10 capsules a day or *PowerGrab* powder formula 1 teaspoon to 1 tablespoon, 5 times a day for 5 days straight, then two days off, repeat as necessary. In the evening, continue to use *PowerPoop* at double the dosage, if not more. The *PowerGrab* bulks up and is a constipating formula to many. Do not be surprised that you are not pooping much when using a formula like *PowerGrab*. It may even be a day or so before you do.

> Note: You did not read the direction wrong; this is a very heavy dose of this formula. You do not want to miss this step. I can attribute the biggest piece of my healing to this formula. This step takes a dedication that might need to be repeated for more than one time.

Results

This procedure may take several weeks to a month before you start seeing results. I took it during a 37-day fast; from Day 16 to Day 37, I had 14 FEET of old, dry, black sludge come out. Your goal is to get the build-up of old, dry fecal matter and excess mucous out of the way. According to Dr. Christopher, you are lucky to be absorbing 3-5% of the nutrients you consume. Once the colon is cleansed you will be absorbing 40-45%.[1] This is where your body will feel the difference in digestion, the colon will work better, and your body will feel better than ever.

HELLO, NUTRIENTS!

---

1   Christopher, John. *Herbal Lectures*, Christopher Publications. Audio CD.
        http://www.christopherpublications.com/Herbal_Lectures_CD.html

2nd Cleansing (Beginner Level) - Gentle Liver Flush

What You Will Need:

- Olive oil
- Juice: grapefruit, orange juice, lemon or lime (This is for your taste preference only)
- *LiverPower Tincture*
- Garlic
- Garlic press
- *DetoxPower Tea*

Each day you will make a drink of fresh juice, garlic, and olive oil. Also drink a cup of *DetoxPower Tea* with a dropperful of the *LiverPower Tincture* to help push the olive oil mixture through you.

During this protocol, you may or may not have a nauseous feeling. If you do, don't be alarmed. It is just an indicator that your liver is constipated. The feeling that I got when I first started doing this was as if I'd had too many alcohol drinks. As you go along with this protocol and the buildup of stones and cholesterol begin moving and releasing, any nauseous feeling will subside.

The rest of the day, consume two more dropperfuls of *LiverPower Tincture* and castor oil pack (Ch. 13) to help stimulate the liver for the following day. Easy way to remember this protocol is 1-2-3-2-1, which is the pattern of changes in olive oil and cloves of garlic each day.

Day 1

Once a day, combine and shake well:
- 1 clove freshly minced garlic
- 1 oz. of olive oil
- 8 oz. fruits, freshly juiced (see recipies in Appendix C)

Three times a day, drink:
- *DetoxPower Tea* with 1 dropperful of *LiverPower*

Day 2

Once a day, combine and shake well:
- 2 cloves freshly minced garlic
- 2 oz. of olive oil
- 8 oz. fruits, freshly juiced

Three times a day, drink:
- *DetoxPower Tea* with 1 dropperful of *LiverPower*

Day 3

Once a day, combine and shake well:
- 3 cloves freshly minced garlic
- 3 oz. of olive oil
- 8 oz. fruits, freshly juiced

Three times a day, drink:
- *DetoxPower Tea* with 1 dropperful of *LiverPower*

Day 4

Once a day, combine and shake well:
- 2 cloves freshly minced garlic
- 2 oz. of olive oil
- 8 oz. fruits, freshly juiced

Three times a day, drink:
- *DetoxPower Tea* with 1 dropperful of *LiverPower*

Day 5

Once a day, combine and shake well:
- 1 clove freshly minced garlic
- 1 oz. of olive oil
- 8 oz. fruits, freshly juiced

Three times a day, drink:
- *DetoxPower Tea* with 1 dropperful of *LiverPower*

2nd (Advanced Level) - PowerHouse Liver Cleanse and Gallbladder Cleanse Flush

When you move into the liver flush, always make sure your colon is going first, because the stones and cholesterol flush out through your colon. If you are constipated in the colon area, it will only back up, and you will not get the results you are wanting.

This recipe is my favorite for a liver/gallbladder flush, as it is over in one day. I have revised it to match what has worked well for me. The original recipe came from

Dr. Hulda Clark and can be found at:
http://curezone.com/cleanse/liver/huldas_recipe.asp

What you will need:

- 1/2 cup Extra Virgin olive oil (= 1.25 dl)
- 3 grapefruits or lemon, use either one or both
  (If you are on PowerHouse Fast or the Mucous –Free Green Diet, this will be the only time you will move from greens, but it is the only thing that will make the olive oil bearable.)
- 4 tablespoons Epsom salts
- *DetoxPower Tea*
- *LiverPower Tincture*
- Pint jar or other lidded cup
- Castor oil pack
- Hot water bottle or heating pad

About Castor Oil Packs

Why Castor Oil Packs? To open up the capillaries and assist in drawing out poisons, hardened mucous, cysts, tumors, or polyps.

How to Make a Castor Oil Pack: Use a natural fabric, such as flannel, wool or cotton. It should be something that you do not care if you see again — cut up an old sheet or rag into the size of 3' x 2'. Soak the fabric with Castor oil and fold up to the size that will fit over the area of your liver. When done, save it for reuse in a Ziploc bag. Refresh with more castor oil with each use.

Why apply heat? Heat helps in penetrating the oil in further. You can use a hot water bottle or if using an electric heating pad have a towel in between the castor oil pack and heating source.

Pre-Flush Preparation

Choose a day that you can rest the following day for the liver/gallbladder cleanse. Take no medicines, vitamins or pills that you can do without. They could prevent your success. If doing this flush while not on a fast, eat lightly until 2pm. If fasting, make your last live juice be at 2 p.m. This allows the bile to build up and develop pressure in the liver. Higher pressure pushes out more stones.

To assist the stimulation of your liver, several times before 2pm add fresh cloves of garlic (as many as you can stand) to your juice; if eating chew them first with your back molars and wash down with water immediately. Garlic you cannot swallow hole otherwise the chemical constituents of garlic will not break lose. Also, before and after drink *DetoxPower Tea* and include a dropperful of *LiverPower Tincture*.

Day 1

Juice the 3 large grapefruits or lemon and mix 4 tbs. of Epsom Salt; pour this into a jar with a lid and shake. This makes 4 servings at 3/4 (three-fourths) cup. Set the jar in the refrigerator to get ice-cold. (This is for convenience and taste only.)

- **2:00 PM.** Do *not* eat or drink after 2 p.m. If you break this rule, you could feel quite ill later. If you are on the PowerHouse Fast, consume your last juice at this time.

- **6:00 PM.** Drink one serving 3/4 (three-fourths) cup of the ice-cold Epsom salt/fruit mixture. You may also drink a few mouthfuls of water afterwards, or rinse your mouth.

- **8:00 PM.** Repeat by drinking another 3/4 (three fourths) cup of the Epsom salt/fruit mixture. You haven't eaten since two o'clock, but you won't feel hungry. Get your bedtime chores done. The timing is critical for success.

- **9:45 PM.** Pour 1/2 (half) cup olive oil into the pint jar and your third dose of the Epsom salts/fruit mixture. Close the jar tightly with the lid and shake hard until watery. (Only fresh grapefruit juice does this.) Now visit the bathroom one or more times, even if it makes you a little late for your ten o'clock drink, but don't be more than 15 minutes late or you will flush fewer stones.

Note: If you didn't consume garlic today or want to add more power to your flush, add Garlic Paste to your feet, as mentioned in Chapter 11.

- **10:00 PM.** Drink the potion you have mixed. Take it all to your bedside if you want, but drink it standing up. Get it down within 5 minutes (fifteen minutes for very elderly or weak persons). The easiest way for me is just to grin and bear it, and shoot it down. Some may use a shake straw.

Lie down immediately. You might fail to get stones out, if you don't. The sooner you lie down, the more stones you will get out. Be ready for bed ahead of time. Don't clean up the kitchen. As soon as the drink is down, walk to your bed and lie down flat on your back with your head up high on the pillow. Try to think about what is happening in the liver. You may feel a train of stones traveling along the bile ducts like marbles. There is no pain because the bile duct valves are open. (Thank you, Epsom Salt!).

Put a castor oil pack over your liver and apply heat over it (hot-water bottle or heating pad), as this will stimulate the liver to function more. Wear an old t-shirt and sleep on an old towel or sheets, as castor oil will stain fabric. Go to sleep now.

Day 2

Next morning, upon awakening, take your fourth and last dose of the Epsom Salt/ fruit mixture. Do not consume this before 6:00 am.

When you awake that morning, the stones will begin dropping out of your colon with a mixture of feces and stones. It can last from the first hour to all day depending on your body and how hard you've tried to do exactly what this says to do.

At times your liver stones, you may be more or less, bigger or smaller. My first liver flush, they were sand size, with more liver flushes they got larger and then smaller again. Just depends how they are inside of you.

Some will use a screen to get the stones. Sound weird? Believe me by this stage you like to discover precisely what is coming out. It is amazing.

You may not feel like consuming much first in the morning hours, and that is normal. Your colon will be moving fragmented pieces of feces from all the Epsom Salt that was consumed from the prior evening. Some will frequent the bathroom for the first few hours in the morning, and it should decrease after that and then return to your usual pattern. Relax today and pat yourself on the back as you see the rewards that come out from all the work you put into this. Later in the morning you are ready to continue on with your day, whether you are fasting or eating.

If you experience indigestion or nausea, it's called a constipated liver and is not allowing the olive oil to move freely through you. Don't worry. The more liver flushes you have accomplished the feeling of nausea will decrease or never happen again.

The first experiences I had with a liver flush; it would have helped to use a castor oil pack. It felt as if I'd had too many drinks of alcohol and the rooms were spinning. This was from the liver being over-constipated.

Remedy for Nausea

Put castor oil pack over the liver, and drink *DetoxPower Tea* with a dropper full of *LiverPower* to help stimulate the liver and move the oil and stones through. Wait until the nausea is gone before drinking the Epsom salt/fruit mixture again. You may go back to bed.

3rd Cleansing – Kidney Flush

This will help release any built-up crystallization of inorganic minerals and salts in your body, and help strengthen and tone your kidneys. A kidney flush can be done many times, and at any time, in a person's life. For the optimum kidney cleanse, use *DetoxPower Tea* and *KidneyPower Formula* at the same time. Herbs are made into a tea and into a tincture because they have some properties and constituents that are water-soluble and others that are best extracted by alcohol. To ensure you receive the most possible from each herb, use both a tea and a tincture. When doing any cleanse or home treatment, one should consult a health professional before beginning.

What you will need

- 3 lemons per day
- 32 ounces of distilled water per day
- *CayennePower Tincture*
- *KidneyPower Tincture*
- *DetoxPower Tea*
- Stevia or maple syrup for sweetness, if needed (omit when on PowerHouse Fast)

Days 1-5

Once a day, combine and shake well:

- Squeeze the juice out of 3 fresh lemons
- Mix with 32 ounces of water
- Add 1 to 3 dropperfuls of *CayennePower*

For five days, drink this mixture daily. Each day, make a new batch. You can drink this warm or cold. You can drink this throughout the day.

Three times a day, drink:

- Drink *DetoxPower Tea* with 1 dropperful of *KidneyPower.*

Optional Fruit Juice*

An excellent diuretic juice that will assist in your kidney flush is made from watermelon. The taste is very pleasant and you won't believe how well it works.

Juice a watermelon, with seeds. Do NOT use seedless. There are a ton of nutrients in those seeds. An ounce of dried watermelon seed kernels contains about 3 grams of zinc (25 percent of the Recommended Dietary Allowance (RDA) for a woman under 50) and 2 grams of iron (14 percent of the RDA). On the minus side, it also contains 158 calories and more than 13 grams of fat.

You will be using the whole watermelon rind, the seeds and the pinkish flesh. There is no waste at all. Cut it up to fit through the hole of your juicing machine. Depending on the size of the watermelon, you may have to cut it in quarters and save the rest for later or eat it. The goal is to get about 12-32 ounces per day.

*Omit watermelon if on the PowerHouse Fast because of its higher carbohydrates.

4ᵗʰ – Blood Flush

This is simple, but critical. Now that you have done all this wonderful work cleansing your organs, it is time to cleanse the blood that flows through them.

You ask, "why make the blood the last of the cleansing?"

When the colon, kidneys, and liver are dilapidated and are unable to filter the debris, they cannot keep the blood clean of waste. Once the organs are cleansed, they are now ready for a high performance of filtering of the inorganic minerals and excess debris in the blood.

Week 1

Three times a day:

- Take 1 dropperful of the *PowerBlood Cleansing Tincture*

If on the 30 day fast, you can start the *PowerBlood Cleansing Tincture* on the last week, even as other cleansings continuing with colon, liver, and kidneys. This was mention in a previous chapter.

CHAPTER 14

BEGINNER – MUCOUS-FREE DIET

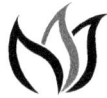

Great news! You CAN overcome illness by taking control with these 3 steps:

"Cleanse, Nourish and Let thy body heal"

Nutrition is a VITAL key to your success. Feed your body what it needs. Hippocrates is famous for saying, "Let food be thy medicine and medicine be thy food."

The Mucous-Free Diet is the diet to help you, from your hooter to your tooter, get back to health. With this diet, you will begin seeing a difference in numerous things immediately, including such health issues as acne, aching muscles, achy joints, and more. This diet works! It is a powerful way to start out if you are unsure about fasting.

The only downside is that it will take a while to get to the finish line for the critically ill. You must not cheat; if you do, it will not work. This diet is not mandatory for the rest of your life. Once you get your body back to optimum health and cleansed out, then your reward is that you will not be as restricted as to what you can consume (Chapter 17 Life After Fasting) or you may stick with this way of eating for the rest of your life. Ideally and realistically, make wholesome foods 80% of eating.

The value of this Mucous-Free diet is it gives your body a break from years of mucous forming foods, and allows your body to focus on what needs to be healed.

Must Have Cookbook

A couple of cookbooks that are a "must have" for vegan cooking are: Veganomicon and Vegan with a Vengeance. Both books are written by Isa Chandra Moskowitz and Terry Hope Romero. These two books will teach you how to prepare a recipe for Ranch dressing that is far superior plus it is medicinal as well, with NO dairy. I bet you are saying, "How can that be?" Check out these books and try it for yourself – you will see.

Cleansing

GREAT news! You can overcome by taking control, eating healthy, and cleansing! Between the ways of eating, you need to work on organ cleansing of the old, stuck, plastered grunge, built up stones, and the constipation of your organs. You have some work ahead of you, your condition being the result of all the years of poor quality foods we all have put into our bodies and other environmental conditions.

The cells of the colon and bacteria in the large intestines have a delicate balance that can easily be destroyed by food, stress, and chemicals in the environment. If your colon and digestive functions are not working well, the body operates in a condition known as auto-intoxication. This means the body is working energetically to rid itself of toxins but cannot keep up. Toxins are recycled, rather than expelled. An out of balance colon may be at the foundation of ailments and diseases from A to Z that has to do with your body.

Here is an analogy to think about: if you had a plugged up toilet would you leave it? Of course not, it would stink! That is what we do with our bodies when we are constipated. It is critical to maintain proper colon function. I cannot stress this enough. It is the number one place to work on first! You will find it affects your body from head-to-toe, young and old, it truly does not matter. Just remember, if it is a cold, a headache, or an incurable disease, the primary area to work on is the colon. Get to POOPING and you'll start seeing results!

My Past Life

Until I started following this healing method, I did not bother buying fresh produce because it would go bad too fast. My thoughts then were, "what a waste of money."

The only fresh produce I received for years were from a salad bar and all vegetables and fruits that I would consume came out of a can. On rare occasion, I purchased frozen produce. I am not much different from many Americans — we like food and like it fast.

Sure, I would make meals for my family, and consistently made out of meat, dairy, and a lot of gluten products such as noodles. Needless to say," ALL MUCOUS FORMING FOODS." I knew nothing about preparing items to their wholesome sprouting state.

Prior to getting sick, I would have to bet it had been several years since I had purchased fresh produce for our home. I was too busy running my business and taking care of my family. It would perish and mold before I ever got to prepare the fresh produce item.

During my childhood, there was never much to speak of for fresh produce. This is the eating habits of how I was raised. I am not blaming and we only do what we know. Looking at the whole picture it is clear, that is how I got so sick in the first place.

Good news, I am living proof of where it is never too late. Let's start now…

What Does This Food From The Earth Do?

Intended for all living beings – it is natural, and it is right here and right now.

It is living food that will supply your body with all of the essential nutrients. It is completely easy and at our fingertips. It sounds too easy to be true, but it is, I am living proof!

If you look at other countries, they are not nearly as sick as we Americans are. They do not suffer like we do, for the straightforward reason that we want our food right now, quickly.

Think, about how much less time it takes to prepare a meal, than to drive to the restaurant, wait in line, wait to be served, eat our meal, and then drive home. You could have been all done. Think about how long it takes to eat out for lunch. A brown sack at home could have already been prepared.

A nutritious meal that would make you feels so much better than if you dine out. Just pay attention, the next time you grab a burger, fries and a Coke; shortly thereafter, you will feel exhausted and groggy.

List of the Do's and Don'ts

Do:

- Eat all the fresh fruits and vegetables you want, raw and lightly steamed. Go all green if you are ready to PowerHouse it!
- Drink all the fresh, live juice you want
- Gallon of distilled water or ½ of your body weight in ounces
- Drink herbal tea
- Use oils (olive oil, wheat germ oil, flax seed oil, coconut oil)
- Cleanse the organs
- Exercise
- Have fun
- Laugh every day

Do but limited:

- Sprouted grains (wheat/gluten)
- Sprouting breads or crackers
- Sprouting nuts and seeds

Don't:

- Eat meat
- Eat dairy, cheese
- Drink dairy
- Eat processed sugar
- Eat processed food
- Consume caffeine
- Consume alcohol

Light at the End of the Tunnel (no, it is not a train!)

The glory in all this — these are not lifetime Do's and Don'ts. It is just until you are feeling better. It is a matter of giving your body a break and feeding it what is very easily digested and processed.

I was never formally diagnosed with Celiac. I could have been if I went to a doctor, to get diagnosed. Celiac disease and wheat and gluten intolerance is on the rise; there will be hearing more and more of this issues from the consumption of the American diet.

I had to keep away from dairy, wheat and gluten products, as they would give my body reaction right after consuming those items. Once this cruddy grunge got out of my system, my body needed all the items of meat, dairy, wheat, and gluten once again. When I continued to eat and added in the item that I stayed away from, my body continued to heal, and I was starved for those items.

Let me explain. These are items that I'd tended to overdose on throughout my life. They work like wallpaper glue and pretty soon my insides did not have very pretty wallpaper on the walls. It was old, dried, and grungy, and nutrients could not blast through that. Once the layer of grunge, was removed from my intestines FREEDOM BEGAN!!!

Mucous-Free Diet Checklist

- Juicer
- Vegetables, fruits, grains, nuts, seeds and legumes
- Garlic
- Water
- Olive Oil
- Lemon
- Distilled Water
- Castor Oil
- Flannel
- Herbal products: *PowerPoop, PowerGrab, DetoxPowerTea, CayennePower, KidneyPower, LiverPower, EchinaceaPower,* and *PowerFood*

Weeks 1 & 3 • Mucous-Free Diet

Note* – Prior to starting, the cleansing procedure get your colon moving. *PowerPoop*, for 2 to 4 weeks.

Day I

LiveJuice & More

- Live Juice, wheatgrass and Mucous-Free Foods all day
- Drink a gallon of distilled water or ½ of your body weight in ounces
- Fresh squeezed lemon ½ of a lemon, 16oz. water and a dropperful of *CayennePower* (or to taste) 3 times a day, hot or cold
- Garlic – juice I clove, three times day
- Hydrotherapy (Ch. 12)
- Skin Brushing (Ch. 12)
- Exercise
- Fresh air and sunlight

Herbal Supplements

- *EchinaceaPower*, I dropperful 3 times a day
- *PowerGrab* 7-10 capsules 5 times a day/ *PowerGrab* Powder I tsp to I tbl 5 times a day
- *PowerFood*, 3 or more capsules 3 times a day
- *DetoxPower Tea*, 3 cups a day
- *KidneyPower*, I dropperful 3 times day
- *PowerPoop*, double dosage of what you were taking for the colon cleansing
- *PowerGrab**

    Note* - This is somewhat constipating; don't be surprised if you don't have a movement all day

Weeks 1 & 3 • Mucous-Free Diet

Day 2

LiveJuice & More

- Live Juice, wheatgrass and Mucous-Free Foods all day
- Drink a gallon of distilled water or ½ of your body weight in ounces
- Fresh squeezed lemon ½ of a lemon, 16oz. water and a dropperful of *CayennePower* (or to taste) 3 times a day, hot or cold
- Garlic – juice 1 clove, three times day
- Hydrotherapy (Ch. 12)
- Skin Brushing (Ch. 12)
- Exercise
- Fresh air and sunlight

Herbal Supplements

- *EchinaceaPower*, 1 dropperful 3 times a day
- *PowerGrab* 7-10 capsules 5 times a day/ *PowerGrab* Powder 1 tsp to 1 tbl 5 times a day
- *PowerFood*, 3 or more capsules 3 times a day
- *DetoxPower Tea*, 3 cups a day
- *KidneyPower*, 1 dropperful 3 times day
- *PowerPoop*, double dosage of what you were taking for the colon cleansing

Weeks 1 & 3 • Mucous-Free Diet

Day 3

LiveJuice & More

- Live Juice, wheatgrass and Mucous-Free Foods all day
- Drink a gallon of distilled water or ½ of your body weight in ounces
- Fresh squeezed lemon ½ of a lemon, 16oz. water and a dropperful *CayennePower* (or to taste) 3 times a day, hot or cold
- Garlic – juice 1 clove, three times day
- Hydrotherapy (Ch. 12)
- Skin Brushing (Ch. 12)
- Exercise
- Fresh air and sunlight

Herbal Supplements

- *EchinaceaPower*, 1 dropperful 3 times a day
- *PowerGrab* 7-10 capsules 5 times a day/ *PowerGrab* Powder 1 tsp to 1 tbl 5 times a day
- *PowerFood*, 3 or more capsules 3 times a day
- *DetoxPower Tea*, 3 cups a day
- *KidneyPower*, 1 dropperful 3 times day
- *PowerPoop*, double dosage of what you were taking for the colon cleansing

Weeks 1 & 3 • Mucous-Free Diet

Day 4

LiveJuice & More

- Live Juice, wheatgrass and Mucous-Free Foods all day
- Drink a gallon of distilled water or ½ of your body weight in ounces
- Fresh squeezed lemon ½ of a lemon, 16oz. water and a dropperful of *CayennePower* (or to taste) 3 times a day, hot or cold
- Garlic – juice I clove, three times day
- Hydrotherapy (Ch. 12)
- Skin Brushing (Ch. 12)
- Exercise
- Fresh air and sunlight

Herbal Supplements

- *EchinaceaPower*, I dropperful 3 times a day
- *PowerGrab* 7-10 capsules 5 times a day/ *PowerGrab* Powder I tsp to I tbl 5 times a day
- *PowerFood*, 3 or more capsules 3 times a day
- *DetoxPower Tea*, 3 cups a day
- *KidneyPower*, I dropperful 3 times day
- *PowerPoop*, double dosage of what you were taking for the colon cleansing

Weeks 1 & 3 • Mucous-Free Diet

Day 5

LiveJuice & More

- Live Juice, wheatgrass and Mucous-Free Foods all day
- Drink a gallon of distilled water or ½ of your body weight in ounces
- Fresh squeezed lemon ½ of a lemon, 16oz. water and a dropperful of *CayennePower* (or to taste) 3 times a day, hot or cold
- Garlic – juice 1 clove, three times day
- Hydrotherapy (Ch. 12)
- Skin Brushing (Ch. 12)
- Exercise
- Fresh air and sunlight

Herbal Supplements

- *EchinaceaPower*, 1 dropperful 3 times a day
- *PowerGrab* 7-10 capsules 5 times a day/ *PowerGrab* Powder 1 tsp to 1 tbl 5 times a day
- *PowerFood*, 3 or more capsules 3 times a day
- *DetoxPower Tea*, 3 cups a day
- *KidneyPower*, 1 dropperful 3 times day
- *PowerPoop*, double dosage of what you were taking for the colon cleansing

Weeks 1 & 3 • Mucous-Free Diet

Day 6

LiveJuice & More

- Live Juice, wheatgrass and Mucous-Free Foods all day
- Drink a gallon of distilled water or ½ of your body weight in ounces
- Fresh squeezed lemon, 16oz. water and a dropperful *CayennePower* (or to taste) 3 times a day, hot or cold
- Garlic – juice 1 clove, three times day
- Hydrotherapy (Ch. 12)
- Skin Brushing (Ch. 12)
- Exercise
- Fresh air and sunlight

Herbal Supplements

- *EchinaceaPower*, 1 dropperful 3 times a day
- *PowerFood*, 3 or more capsules 3 times a day
- *DetoxPower Tea*, 3 cups a day, 3 times a day
- *KidneyPower*, 1 dropperful 3 times day
- *PowerPoop*, you are done with the 5 days of *PowerGrab*. You don't have to take extra of the *PowerPoop* today, unless needed

Weeks 1 & 3 • Mucous-Free Diet

Day 7

LiveJuice & More

- Day of rest, you will not take any herbal supplements
- Live Juice, wheatgrass and Mucous-Free Foods all day
- Drink a gallon of distilled water or ½ of your body weight in ounces
- Colonics or high enema (Ch. 12)

Weeks 2 & 4 • Mucous-Free Diet

Day 1

LiveJuice & More

- Live Juice, wheatgrass and Mucous-Free Foods all day
- Fresh squeezed lemon, 16oz. water and a dropperful *CayennePower* (or to taste) 3 times a day, hot or cold
- Drink a gallon of distilled water or ½ of your body weight in ounces
- Hydrotherapy (Ch. 12)
- Skin Brushing (Ch. 12)
- Exercise
- Fresh air and sunlight

Herbal Supplements

- *EchinaceaPower*, 1 dropperful 3 times a day
- *LiverPower*, 1 dropperful 3 times day + Gentle liver Flush
- *PowerFood*, 3 or more capsules 3 times a day
- *DetoxPower Tea*, 3 cups a day
- *PowerPoop*, same dosage as during colon flush
- Castor Oil Pack each evening at least for 2 hours (I prefer to go to bed with the castor pack on)

Weeks 2 & 4 • Mucous-Free Diet

Day 2

LiveJuice & More

- Live Juice, wheatgrass and Mucous-Free Foods all day
- Fresh squeezed lemon, 16oz. water and a dropperful *CayennePower* (or to taste) 3 times a day, hot or cold
- Drink a gallon of distilled water or ½ of your body weight in ounces
- Hydrotherapy (Ch. 12)
- Skin Brushing (Ch. 12)
- Exercise
- Fresh air and sunlight

Herbal Supplements

- *EchinaceaPower*, 1 dropperful 3 times a day
- *LiverPower*, 1 dropperful 3 times day plus Gentle Liver Flush
- *PowerFood*, 3 or more capsules 3 times a day
- *DetoxPower Tea*, 3 cups a day
- *PowerPoop*, same dosage as during colon flush
- Castor Oil Pack each evening at least for 2 hours (I prefer to go to bed with it on)

Weeks 2 & 4 • Mucous-Free Diet

Day 3

LiveJuice & More

- Live Juice, wheatgrass and Mucous-Free Foods all day
- Fresh squeezed lemon, 16oz. water and a dropperful *CayennePower* (or to taste) 3 times a day, hot or cold
- Drink a gallon of distilled water or ½ of your body weight in ounces
- Hydrotherapy (Ch. 12)
- Skin Brushing (Ch. 12)
- Exercise
- Fresh air and sunlight

Herbal Supplements

- *EchinaceaPower*, 1 dropperful 3 times a day
- *LiverPower*, 1 dropperful 3 times day plus Gentle liver Flush
- *PowerFood*, 3 or more capsules 3 times a day
- *DetoxPower Tea*, 3 cups a day
- *PowerPoop*, same dosage as during colon flush
- Castor Oil Pack each evening at least for 2 hours (I prefer to go to bed with it on)

Weeks 2 & 4 • Mucous-Free Diet

Day 4

LiveJuice & More

- Live Juice, wheatgrass and Mucous-Free Foods all day
- Fresh squeezed lemon, 16oz. water and a dropperful *CayennePower* (or to taste) 3 times a day, hot or cold
- Drink a gallon of distilled water or ½ of your body weight in ounces
- Hydrotherapy (Ch. 12)
- Skin Brushing (Ch. 12)
- Exercise
- Fresh air and sunlight

Herbal Supplements

- *EchinaceaPower*, 1 dropperful 3 times a day
- *LiverPower*, 1 dropperful 3 times day plus Gentle Liver Flush
- *PowerFood*, 3 or more capsules 3 times a day
- *DetoxPower Tea*, 3 cups a day
- *PowerPoop*, same dosage as during colon flush
- Castor Oil Pack each evening at least for 2 hours (I prefer to go to bed with it on)

Weeks 2 & 4 • Mucous-Free Diet

Day 5

LiveJuice & More

- Live Juice, wheatgrass and Mucous-Free Foods all day
- Fresh squeezed lemon, 16oz. water and a dropperful *CayennePower* (or to taste) 3 times a day, hot or cold
- Drink a gallon of distilled water or ½ of your body weight in ounces
- Hydrotherapy (Ch. 12)
- Skin Brushing (Ch. 12)
- Exercise
- Fresh air and sunlight

Herbal Supplements

- *EchinaceaPower*, 1 dropperful 3 times a day
- *LiverPower*, 1 dropperful 3 times day plus Gentle Liver Flush
- *PowerFood*, 3 or more capsules 3 times a day
- *DetoxPower Tea*, 3 cups a day
- *PowerPoop*, same dosage as during colon flush
- Castor Oil Pack each evening at least for 2 hours (I prefer to go to bed with it on)

Weeks 2 & 4 • Mucous-Free Diet

Day 6

LiveJuice & More

- Live Juice, wheatgrass and Mucous-Free Foods all day
- Fresh squeezed lemon, 16oz. water and a dropperful *CayennePower* (or to taste) 3 times a day, hot or cold
- Drink a gallon of distilled water or ½ of your body weight in ounces
- Hydrotherapy (Ch. 12)
- Skin Brushing (Ch. 12)
- Exercise
- Fresh air and sunlight

Herbal Supplements

- *EchinaceaPower*, 1 dropperful 3 times a day
- *PowerPoop*, same dosage as during colon flush
- *PowerFood*, 3 or more capsules 3 times a day
- *DetoxPower Tea*, 3 cups a day

Weeks 2 & 4 • Mucous-Free Diet

Day 7

LiveJuice & More

- Day of rest, you will not take any herbal supplements
- Live Juice, wheatgrass and Mucous-Free Foods all day
- Drink a gallon of distilled water or ½ of your body weight in ounces
- Colonics or high enema (Ch. 12)

The last 7 days of a 30 day cleanse, add in *BloodCleansing Power Tincture* for 3 times a day and use this for 6 days on and 1 day off, for a total of 3 weeks. Continue after the 30 day cleansing protocol is over.

CHAPTER 15

INTERMEDIATE – JUICEPOWER FAST

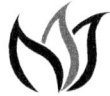

With the JuicePower fast you have the freedom of making all the flavorful live juices. This particular fast got me out of rocky waters many times. There is a lot power in JuicePower fasting.

When you follow this, you can do more of the juices I prefer. I like to think of myself as the Paula Deen of juicing. NOOO, I never put a cake in the juicer!

This protocol is very valuable. You may remember reading in my story how this saved me at the beginning, and it can save you too. I always tried to make everything taste good. It was a good way to get started and the fasts were beneficial but not enough for the full healing I needed. My body had such an issue with Candida that I had use the PowerHouse Fast until the yeast overgrowth was under control. If you find the healing benefits from this fast are short-lived, then move on to the PowerHouse Fast.

You will be amazed to discover how rewarding and simple this works. Ailments you have become so accustomed too, start to disappear. All thanks to your dedicated work of the JuicePower fast.

It's Powerful. "Keep your eye on the prize."

Main Aim of JuicePower Fasting

1. Rid yourself of the old stuck debris in your organs so your body has the ability to assume and assimilate nutrients. This also helps the filters of your body so they can work properly.

2. Blast your body full of nutrients

FAQs About the JuicePower Fast

Q: Can I make my vegetable juice in the morning and drink it later in the day?

A: It is much better than not drinking any at all. Live juice is ideal when drank immediately. Live juice is one of the most perishable foods.

However, if you are careful, you can store your live juice in a sealed glass container for up to 24 hours with a moderate nutritional decline. Filling it to the top of the jar, so there is little room for extra air that will oxidize and damage your juice.

Think of a cut or bitten apple turning brown when exposed to air.

Use an opaque container to block out all light, and then store it in the refrigerator until 30 minutes prior to drinking. Ideally the juice should be consumed at room temperature.

Q: What type of vegetables should I juice?

A: Here are excellent introduction combos for the beginner:

Beet + fennel + carrots + apple

Carrot + apple+ ginger root

Once you get used to these live juices, you can start adding the produce that is less palatable but more nutritional and has more chlorophyll. Green vegetables have the most value to use in your vegetable juicing program.

For starters, the green vegetables to include in your juicing are lettuces. You can then put in some of the other similar green leafy vegetables such as spinach, kale, and cabbage. Cabbage juice is one of the most healing juices when it comes to repairing an ulcer and a good source of vitamins.

Herbs also make marvelous combinations such as ginger root, fennel, parsley, cilantro, garlic and you will find many more.

You will find more recipes in Appendix C.

Q: What about wheatgrass?

A: Wheatgrass is an excellent shot of juice. One ounce of wheatgrass is so powerful it is equivalent to 10 pounds of vegetables.

Q: What about the taste?

A: One main objection people raise when trying the taste of live juicing is the taste. They cannot stand it. There is a solution. For this JuicePower Fast, I recommend adding few seedless grapes or apples in your vegetable juice. It has a great way to improving the taste of your juice. In the more vegetable flavored juices add CayennePower to the juice, it will cut the taste of greens.

Q: Should I use only one recipe?

A: Chances are quite high that if you keep juicing the same vegetables and fruits for any length of time you will become allergic to them. Variety is the spice of life.

Q: I can't take another drink of olive oil; I threw up the last time or it made me extremely nauseous!

A: Get a better tasting olive oil, such as the brand Chiara. Your liver is constipated and the more you do liver flushes that will subside.

Q: My body is getting weak from water!

A: You need more nutrition, get to juicing.

Q: What kind of salt should I use and how much?

A: Sea salt is best: highest mineral content. Use a measuring teaspoon. The rule of thumb is 1/8 teaspoon for every 16 oz.; 1/4 teaspoon for every 32 oz (1 quart); 1/2 teaspoon for 64 oz., or 1 full teaspoon for 1 gallon. (Some people will need less salt, others more). This is a starting point, not a set rule. You can just add the salt to your food or add the salt to the water and shake or stir it. The best way is to just throw the salt into your mouth and chase it with water.

Q: What if my body swells from consuming salt?

A: If your ankles, fingers, or eyelids swell, don't do the salt for two days, just drink the water. Then on the 3rd day begin taking the salt again.

NOTE: If your kidneys are not working well, then don't follow this program. If you still want to try it on your own, just drink one eight-ounce glass of water and wait until you go to the bathroom. Then drink another glass. When your kidneys come up to speed (input matches output), then start the salt slowly to make sure your kidneys are working ok. Always consult with your health care provider.

Couple Of Adjustments You Can Make

1. JuicePower fast version, you can do the Gentle Liver Flush or PowerHouse Liver/Gallbladder Flush. In this 4-week schedule, I have only listed two Gentle Liver Flushes, if you find the need do more, then do more. I did the PowerHouse Liver Flush once a week during the 37 day fast.

2. Some days you may feel all you want to do is drink water. That is okay. As you may recall, I made it ten solids days in a row on water only during the 37 day fast. During that time, I still took the herbal supplements, as I did not stop working on cleansing my organs.

3. I typically start *PowerGrab* on Mondays, so it is a no brainier for me to re-member since the *PowerGrab* is only for 5 days, and then give it a two-day break.

Must Have Checklist

- Juicing Machine
- Vegetables, fruits and wheatgrass
- Garlic
- Water
- Olive Oil (I prefer Chiara brand; it is wrapped with gold foil)
- Lemon, Lime or Grapefruit for the liver flush
- Epsom Salts
- Distilled Water
- Castor Oil
- Flannel
- My herbal supplements: *PowerPoop, PowerGrab, DetoxPower Tea, CayennePower, KidneyPower, LiverPower, EchinaceaPower* and *PowerFood*

Weeks 1 & 3 • JuicePower Fast

*NOTE: Prior to starting any cleansing protocol, have your colon moving by taking *PowerPoop* for 2 to 4 weeks. Flushing will be much more effective if there isn't much blockage. You can also do more enemas while cleansing then what is discussed.

Day 1

LiveJuice & More

- Live Juice of your choice and wheatgrass
- Drink a gallon of distilled water
- Fresh squeezed lemon ½ of a lemon, 16oz. water and a dropperful of *CayennePower* (or to taste) 3 times a day, hot or cold
- Garlic – juice 1 clove, 3 times a day
- Hydrotherapy (Ch. 12)
- Skin Brushing (Ch. 12)
- Exercise
- Fresh air and sunlight

Herbal Supplements

- *EchinaceaPower*, 1 dropperful 3 times a day
- *PowerGrab* 7-10 capsules 5 times a day/ *PowerGrab* Powder 1 tsp to 1 tbl 5 times a day

  Note: *PowerGrab* is somewhat constipating; don't be surprised if you don't have a movement all day
- *PowerFood*, 3 or more capsules 3 times a day
- *DetoxPower Tea*, 3 cups a day
- *KidneyPower*, 1 dropperful 3 times day
- *PowerPoop*, double dosage of what you were taking for the colon cleansing

Weeks 1 & 3 • JuicePower Fast

Day 2

LiveJuice & More

- Live Juice of your choice and wheatgrass
- Drink a gallon of distilled water or ½ of your body weight in ounces
- Fresh squeezed lemon ½ of a lemon, 16oz. water and a dropperful of *CayennePower* (or to taste) 3 times a day, hot or cold
- Garlic – juice 1 clove, 3 times a day
- Hydrotherapy (Ch. 12)
- Skin Brushing (Ch. 12)
- Exercise
- Fresh air and sunlight

Herbal Supplements

- *EchinaceaPower*, 1 dropperful 3 times a day
- *PowerGrab* 7-10 capsules 5 times a day/ *PowerGrab* Powder 1 tsp to 1 tbl 5 times a day
- *PowerFood*, 3 or more capsules 3 times a day
- *DetoxPower Tea*, 3 cups a day
- *KidneyPower*, 1 dropperful 3 times day
- *PowerPoop*, double dosage of what you were taking for the colon cleansing

Weeks 1 & 3 • JuicePower Fast

Day 3

LiveJuice & More

- Live Juice of your choice and wheatgrass
- Drink a gallon of distilled water or ½ of your body weight in ounces
- Fresh squeezed lemon ½ of a lemon, 16oz. water and a dropperful of *CayennePower* (or to taste) 3 times a day, hot or cold
- Garlic – juice 1 clove, 3 times a day
- Hydrotherapy (Ch. 12)
- Skin Brushing (Ch. 12)
- Exercise
- Fresh air and sunlight

Herbal Supplements

- *EchinaceaPower*, 1 dropperful 3 times a day
- *PowerGrab* 7-10 capsules 5 times a day/ *PowerGrab* Powder 1 tsp to 1 tbl 5 times a day
- *PowerFood*, 3 or more capsules 3 times a day
- *DetoxPower Tea*, 3 cups a day
- *KidneyPower*, 1 dropperful 3 times day
- *PowerPoop*, double dosage of what you were taking for the colon cleansing

Weeks 1 & 3 • JuicePower Fast

Day 4

LiveJuice & More

- Live Juice of your choice and wheatgrass
- Drink a gallon of distilled water or ½ of your body weight in ounces
- Fresh squeezed lemon ½ of a lemon, 16oz. water and a dropperful of *CayennePower* (or to taste) 3 times a day, hot or cold
- Garlic – juice 1 clove, 3 times a day
- Hydrotherapy (Ch. 12)
- Skin Brushing (Ch. 12)
- Exercise
- Fresh air and sunlight

Herbal Supplements

- *EchinaceaPower*, 1 dropperful 3 times a day
- *PowerGrab* 7-10 capsules 5 times a day/ *PowerGrab* Powder 1 tsp to 1 tbl 5 times a day
- *PowerFood*, 3 or more capsules 3 times a day
- *DetoxPower Tea*, 3 cups a day
- *KidneyPower*, 1 dropperful 3 times day
- *PowerPoop*, double dosage of what you were taking for the colon cleansing

Weeks 1 & 3 • JuicePower Fast

Day 5

LiveJuice & More

- Live Juice of your choice and wheatgrass
- Drink a gallon of distilled water or ½ of your body weight in ounces
- Fresh squeezed lemon ½ of a lemon, 16oz. water and a dropperful of *CayennePower* (or to taste) 3 times a day, hot or cold
- Garlic – juice 1 clove, 3 times a day
- Hydrotherapy (Ch. 12)
- Skin Brushing (Ch. 12)
- Exercise
- Fresh air and sunlight

Herbal Supplements

- *EchinaceaPower*, 1 dropperful 3 times a day
- *PowerGrab* 7-10 capsules 5 times a day/ *PowerGrab* Powder 1 tsp to 1 tbl 5 times a day
- *PowerFood*, 3 or more capsules 3 times a day
- *DetoxPower Tea*, 3 cups a day
- *KidneyPower*, 1 dropperful 3 times day
- *PowerPoop*, double dosage of what you were taking for the colon cleansing

Weeks 1 & 3 • JuicePower Fast

Day 6

LiveJuice & More

- Live Juice of your choice and wheatgrass
- Drink a gallon of distilled water or ½ of your body weight in ounces
- Fresh squeezed lemon, 16oz. water and a dropperful *CayennePower* (or to taste) 3 times a day, hot or cold
- Garlic – juice 1 clove, 3 times a day
- Hydrotherapy (Ch. 12)
- Skin Brushing (Ch. 12)
- Exercise
- Fresh air and sunlight

Herbal Supplements

- *EchinaceaPower*, 1 dropperful 3 times a day
- *PowerFood*, 3 or more capsules 3 times a day
- *DetoxPower Tea*, 3 cups a day, 3 times a day
- *KidneyPower*, 1 dropperful 3 times day
- *PowerPoop* – you are done with the 5 days of *PowerGrab* and do not have to take extra of the *PowerPoop* today unless needed

Weeks 1 & 3 • JuicePower Fast

Day 7

LiveJuice & More

- Day of rest, you will not take any herbal supplements
- Live Juice of your choice and wheatgrass
- Drink a gallon of distilled water
- Colonics or high enema (Ch. 12)

Weeks 2 & 4 • JuicePower Fast

Day 1

LiveJuice & More

- Live Juice of your choice and wheatgrass
- Fresh squeezed lemon, 16oz. water and a dropperful *CayennePower* (or to taste) 3 times a day, hot or cold
- Drink a gallon of distilled water or ½ of your body weight in ounces
- Hydrotherapy (Ch. 12)
- Skin Brushing (Ch. 12)
- Exercise
- Fresh air and sunlight

Herbal Supplements

- *EchinaceaPower,* 1 dropperful 3 times a day
- *LiverPower,* 1 dropperful, 3 times day + Gentle Liver Flush
- *PowerFood,* 3 or more, 3 times a day
- *DetoxPower Tea,* 3 cups a day
- *PowerPoop,* same dosage as during colon flush

Weeks 2 & 4 • JuicePower Fast

Day 2

LiveJuice & More

- Live Juice of your choice and wheatgrass
- Fresh squeezed lemon, 16oz. water and a dropperful *CayennePower* (or to taste) 3 times a day, hot or cold
- Drink a gallon of distilled water or ½ of your body weight in ounces
- Hydrotherapy (Ch. 12)
- Skin Brushing (Ch. 12)
- Exercise
- Fresh air and sunlight

Herbal Supplements

- *EchinaceaPower*, 1 dropperful 3 times a day
- *LiverPower*, 1 dropperful, 3 times day + Gentle Liver Flush (Ch. 12)
- *PowerFood*, 3 or more, 3 times a day
- *DetoxPower Tea*, 3 cups a day
- *PowerPoop*, same dosage as during colon flush

Weeks 2 & 4 • JuicePower Fast

Day 3

LiveJuice & More

- Live Juice of your choice and wheatgrass
- Fresh squeezed lemon, 16oz. water and a dropperful *CayennePower* (or to taste) 3 times a day, hot or cold
- Drink a gallon of distilled water
- Hydrotherapy (Ch. 12)
- Skin Brushing (Ch. 12)
- Exercise
- Fresh air and sunlight

Herbal Supplements

- *EchinaceaPower,* 1 dropperful 3 times a day
- *LiverPower,* 1 dropperful 3 times day + Gentle Liver Flush (Ch. 12)
- *PowerFood,* 3 or more capsules 3 times a day
- *DetoxPower Tea,* 3 cups a day
- *PowerPoop,* same dosage as during colon flush

Weeks 2 & 4 • JuicePower Fast

Day 4

LiveJuice & More

- Live Juice of your choice and wheatgrass
- Fresh squeezed lemon, 16oz. water and a dropperful *CayennePower* (or to taste) 3 times a day, hot or cold
- Drink a gallon of distilled water or ½ of your body weight in ounces
- Hydrotherapy (Ch. 12)
- Skin Brushing (Ch. 12)
- Exercise
- Fresh air and sunlight

Herbal Supplements

- *EchinaceaPower*, 1 dropperful 3 times a day
- *LiverPower*, 1 dropperful 3 times day + Gentle Liver Flush
- *PowerFood*, 3 or more capsules 3 times a day
- *DetoxPower Tea*, 3 cups a day
- *PowerPoop*, same dosage as during colon flush

Weeks 2 & 4 • JuicePower Fast

Day 5

LiveJuice & More

- Live Juice of your choice and wheatgrass
- Fresh squeezed lemon, 16oz. water and a dropperful *CayennePower* (or to taste) 3 times a day, hot or cold
- Drink a gallon of distilled water or ½ of your body weight in ounces
- Hydrotherapy (Ch. 12)
- Skin Brushing (Ch. 12)
- Exercise
- Fresh air and sunlight

Herbal Supplements

- *EchinaceaPower*, 1 dropperful 3 times a day
- *LiverPower*, 1 dropperful 3 times day + Gentle Liver Flush
- *PowerFood*, 3 or more capsules 3 times a day
- *DetoxPower Tea*, 3 cups a day
- *PowerPoop*, same dosage as during colon flush

Weeks 2 & 4 • JuicePower Fast

Day 6

LiveJuice & More

- Live Juice of your choice and wheatgrass
- Fresh squeezed lemon, 16oz. water and a dropperful *CayennePower* (or to taste) 3 times a day, hot or cold
- Drink a gallon of distilled water or ½ of your body weight in ounces
- Hydrotherapy (Ch. 12)
- Skin Brushing (Ch. 12)
- Exercise
- Fresh air and sunlight

Herbal Supplements

- *EchinaceaPower,* 1 dropperful 3 times a day
- *PowerFood,* 3 or more capsules 3 times a day
- *DetoxPower Tea,* 3 cups a day
- *PowerPoop,* same dosage as during colon flush

Weeks 2 & 4 • JuicePower Fast

Day 7

LiveJuice & More

- Day of rest, you will not take any herbal supplements
- Live Juice of your choice and wheatgrass
- Drink a gallon of distilled water or ½ of your body weight in ounces
- Colonics or high enema (Ch. 12)
- The last 7 day of the 30 day cleanse, add in *BloodCleansing Power Tincture* for 3 times a day and use this for 6 days on and 1 day off, for a total of 3 weeks. Continue after the fasting is over.

CHAPTER 16

ADVANCED – POWERHOUSE FAST HEALING PROGRAM

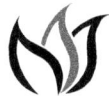

When there is no time to waste, follow these protocols for the PowerHouse Fast. You must be more aggressive than your disease. PowerHouse Fast is the route to follow. These protocols I have written will teach you and help you take control of your individual health with no confusion.

Too many people become health-food-store poor and get nowhere. Sound familiar?

Once you are willing to stop catering to your taste buds for a month, this fast will work for you and work well. Initially, many of us are going to find these juices do not please our taste buds as we have currently developed them. This is where you choose health. You have to be more aggressive than the disease or it will win. You have to do it all, not half, or you will only receive partial or short-term healing, and I know that you want to be strong and healthy again!

Missing Link

My signature PowerHouse fast does not beat around the bush or lollygag around; it will get down to business with improving your health. It will not take years, or even months and has long term results.

When I was first doing "healthy" remedies, you name it, I tried it! I always ended up returning to fasting. My biggest frustration was the benefits did not last...until my PowerHouse Fast.

Often there is a missing link when putting all the pieces of the pie together for natural healing. Very simply:

1. Cleanse
2. Nourish
3. Let Thy Body Heal Itself.

The answer I had been looking for and have provided for you here, is the vital combination of organ cleansing remove all the junk and debris, AND rigorous fasting with exceptionally nutritious juices to nourish the body COMBINED with time to allow the body to heal years of damage in just weeks.

This protocol finally took me to the place where I wanted to be: full and lasting health. PowerHouse fast works, but you must adhere to it rigorously.

Main Aim

- Balance out the overgrowth of Candida, parasites
- Seal a leaky gut
- Rid yourself of the old stuck debris in your organs.

Juicing Low Carb Vegetables

What you will be consuming will not cater to Candida or parasites. They hunger after sweet items. You can have all the GREEN vegetable juice you want, the vegetables that are low carbohydrate and nutritious. Feel free to add in herbs for flavor. Most herbs have little to no carbohydrates.

Greens are not the most appealing taste; at times we have to do what we do not like. This is when you have to ask yourself, "Do you like being sick? " When your answer is "no" then you can use that desire to bolster your will-power and stay on course.

In the beginning, dilute the green juice with water. As you get used to it, dilute it less.

While higher carbohydrate vegetables and fruits, such as the carrots, beets, apples, etc. are generally great for you, they are not what you need right now. All those carbs are not helpful to an ailing body. Once you ridding yourself of contaminates in your body through the PowerHouse Fast, you will be able to re-introduce the higher carbohydrate produce into your diet.

How Long?

In the PowerHouse fast, the longer one goes more lasting healing you will receive. The suggestion is to go 30 days. One round of this fasting may be enough, or possibly you will find later you need to repeat another 30 days to achieve all the results you desire. It is equally possible that two weeks may be enough for you. Just listen to your body, you will know.

You may come up with some ideas of your own, but do not remove yourself far from this schedule. Just remember that I have done every fast that I could get my hands on. Until I followed this protocol of getting all the organs cleansed and all the nutrition that my body needed, I did not receive all the health and vitality that I have today. I know you can have the same too!

Cost

You will spend less than what you spend on eating for the month and have a lot to show for it. I call this a savings, and you will have your health!

This protocol does not care whether you are rich or poor, educated or uneducated. This method is inexpensive but very effective. You are looking at a cost for a month, roughly $300, which will include your vegetables and herbal supplements and the onetime expense of a juice machine ($60-250).

The other cost that can add up is colonics. If cannot afford them, just do the high enema yourself. The enema kits that sell online range from, $8.50 to $225. The wide range in price reflects features such as bag material, bag capacity, choices in accessories, and durability.

Garlic

Garlic is a powerful and vital herb that will speed your recovery. Remember to include it in your recipes. A full explanation of the health benefits mentioned in Chapter 11.

Check List for What You Need

- Juicing machine
- Green vegetables, organic when possible
- Wheatgrass fresh or frozen
- Garlic
- Olive Oil (I prefer Chiara brand, which is wrapped with gold foil)
- Lemon, lime, and grapefruit
- Epsom salts
- Distilled water
- Castor oil
- Flannel
- Heating pad or bottle
- Enema bag

Herbal Supplements

- *PowerPoop, PowerGrab,* DetoxPower, *CayennePower, KidneyPower, LiverPower, PowerFood,* Blood Power Cleanser

PowerGreen Juice

Preferably organic green vegetables, made into live juice. If the green drink is too much for you, in terms of bitterness and strong flavor, you can dilute it with water. That may be more bearable for some. Start with the glass 1/4 full of greens, and the rest filled with distilled water. The next time, fill the glass 1/2 full with greens, and then fill the remaining space with distilled water. Keep upping it from there until you have a glass filled with greens only. Green vegetables have the fewest number of carbs and the most chlorophyll, which helps with the cleansing process.

> *HINT - My favorite to give the greens a better taste is to give it a wham-bam with *CayennePower*! You add as much as you like according to your taste buds

Water

I prefer distilled water; the reason being that distilled water is 'thirsty' water that will help grab the inorganic minerals and salts in your body. Our body consists of 80% fluids, and you need to replenish it daily. When focusing on cleansing out your body, each day drink a gallon of water. The more scientific way; take your body weight number and divide it by 2. That number is how many ounces you should drink a day.

Example: If you weigh 100lbs, then you should drink 50 ounces a day.

I have fasted, with water alone, for 10 days. At the beginning, I thought, I was going to die on water alone; 5 years later I am still here to tell you the story.

Sea Salt

Sea salt is best: highest mineral content. Use a measuring teaspoon. The rule of thumb is 1/8 teaspoon for every 16 oz.; 1/4 teaspoon for every 32 oz (1 quart); 1/2 teaspoon for 64 oz., or 1 full teaspoon for 1 gallon. (Some people will need less salt, others more). This is a starting point, not a set rule. You can just add the salt to your food or add the salt to the water and shake or stir it. The best way is to just throw the salt into your mouth and chase it with water.

Exceptions

The only time you would use a produce that is not green is for the Kidney and Liver/Gallbladder flushes. The lemon, lime, and grapefruit do turn alkaline once they hit your gut and mix with your digestive juices.

PowerHouse Healing Schedule

*NOTE: If time permits your cleansing process will be much more effective, when you start working on your colon prior to embarking on this protocol. Take *PowerPoop* for 2 to 4 weeks. Also, use the enemas if needed.

Day 1

LiveJuice & More

- Green Live Juice and wheatgrass all day
- Drink a gallon of distilled water or ½ of your body weight in ounces
- Fresh squeezed lemon, 16oz. water and a dropperful *CayennePower* (or to taste) 3 times a day, hot or cold
- Garlic – juice 1 clove, 3 times a day
- Hydrotherapy (Ch. 12)
- Skin Brushing (Ch. 12)
- Exercise
- Fresh air and sunlight

Herbal Supplements

- *EchinaceaPower* dropperful, 3 times a day
- *KidneyPower*, 1 dropperful 3 times day
- *PowerFood*, 3 or more capsules 3 times a day
- *DetoxPower Tea*, 3 cups a day
- *LiverPower*, 1 dropperful 3 times day
- *PowerGrab*, 7-10 capsules 5 times a day/ *PowerGrab* Powder 1 tsp to 1 tbl 5 times a day.

   Note: *PowerGrab* is somewhat constipating; don't be surprised if you don't have a movement all day

- *PowerPoop*, double-up to what you didn't take on the fast and as this week progresses you may need to take a few more than the double up.

Weeks 1 & 3 • PowerHouse Fast

Day 2

LiveJuice & More

- Green Live Juice and wheatgrass all day
- Fresh squeezed lemon, 16oz. water and a dropperful *CayennePower* (or to taste) 3 times a day, hot or cold
- Garlic – juice 1 clove, 3 times a day
- Drink a gallon of distilled water or ½ of your body weight in ounces
- Hydrotherapy (Ch. 12)
- Skin Brushing (Ch. 12)
- Exercise
- Fresh air and sunlight

Herbal Supplements

- *EchinaceaPower* dropperful, 3 times a day
- *PowerGrab* 7-10 capsules 5 times a day/ *PowerGrab* Powder 1 tsp to 1 tbl 5 times a day
- *PowerFood*, 3 or more capsules 3 times a day
- *DetoxPower Tea*, 3 cups a day
- *LiverPower*, 1 dropperful 3 times day
- *KidneyPower*, 1 dropperful 3 times day
- *PowerPoop*, double-up

Weeks 1 & 3 • PowerHouse Fast

Day 3

LiveJuice & More

- Green Live Juice and wheatgrass all day
- Drink a gallon of distilled water
- Fresh squeezed lemon, 16oz. water and a dropperful *CayennePower* (or to taste) 3 times a day, hot or cold
- Garlic – juice 1 clove, 3 times a day
- Hydrotherapy (Ch. 12)
- Skin Brushing (Ch. 12)
- Exercise
- Fresh air and sunlight

Herbal Supplements

- *EchinaceaPower* dropperful, 3 times a day
- *PowerGrab* 7-10 capsules 5 times a day/ *PowerGrab* Powder 1 tsp to 1 tbl 5 times a day
- *PowerFood*, 3 or more capsules 3 times a day
- *DetoxPower Tea*, 3 cups a day
- *KidneyPower*, 1 dropperful 3 times day
- *LiverPower*, 1 dropperful 3 times day
- *PowerPoop*, double-up

Weeks 1 & 3 • PowerHouse Fast

Day 4

LiveJuice & More

- Green Live Juice and wheatgrass all day
- Drink a gallon of distilled water or ½ of your body weight in ounces
- Fresh squeezed lemon, 16oz. water and a dropperful *CayennePower* (or to taste) 3 times a day, hot or cold
- Garlic – juice 1 clove, 3 times a day
- Hydrotherapy (Ch. 12)
- Skin Brushing (Ch. 12)
- Exercise
- Fresh air and sunlight

Herbal Supplements

- *EchinaceaPower* dropperful, 3 times a day
- *PowerGrab* 7-10 capsules 5 times a day/ *PowerGrab* Powder 1 tsp to 1 tbl 5 times a day
- *PowerFood*, 3 or more capsules 3 times a day
- *DetoxPower Tea*, 3 cups a day
- *KidneyPower*, 1 dropperful 3 times day
- *LiverPower*, 1 dropperful 3 times day
- *PowerPoop*, double-up

Weeks 1 & 3 • PowerHouse Fast

Day 5

LiveJuice & More

- Green Live Juice and wheatgrass all day
- Drink a gallon of distilled water or ½ of your body weight in ounces
- Fresh squeezed lemon, 16oz. water and a dropperful *CayennePower* (or to taste) 3 times a day, hot or cold
- Garlic – juice 1 clove, 3 times a day
- Hydrotherapy (Ch. 12)
- Skin Brushing (Ch. 12)
- Exercise
- Fresh air and sunlight

Herbal Supplements

- *EchinaceaPower* dropperful, 3 times a day
- *PowerGrab* 7-10 capsules 5 times a day/ *PowerGrab* Powder 1 tsp to 1 tbl 5 times a day
- *PowerFood*, 3 or more capsules 3 times a day
- *DetoxPower Tea*, 3 cups a day
- *LiverPower*, 1 dropperful 3 times day
- *KidneyPower*, 1 dropperful 3 times day
- *PowerPoop*, double-up

Weeks 1 & 3 • PowerHouse Fast

Day 6

LiveJuice & More

- Green Live Juice and wheatgrass till 2 pm
- Drink a gallon of distilled water or ½ of your body weight in ounces
- Fresh squeezed lemon, 16oz. water and a dropperful *CayennePower* (or to taste) 3 times a day, hot or cold
- Consume raw garlic in your juices today, at least 10 cloves. This will help in assisting the liver for the liver flush tonight.
- Hydrotherapy (Ch. 12)
- Skin Brushing (Ch. 12)
- Exercise
- Fresh air and sunlight

Herbal Supplements

- *EchinaceaPower* dropperful, 3 times a day
- *PowerFood*, 3 or more capsules 3 times a day
- *DetoxPower Tea*, 3 cups a day
- *LiverPower*, 1 dropperful 3 times day
- *KidneyPower*, 1 dropperful 3 times day
- PowerHouse Liver Flush (Ch. 13)

Weeks 1 & 3 • PowerHouse Fast

Day 7

LiveJuice & More

- Day of rest, you will not take any herbal supplements
- Green Live Juice and wheatgrass all day
- Drink a gallon of distilled water or ½ of your body weight in ounces
- Colonics or high enema (Ch. 12)

Weeks 2 & 4 • PowerHouse Fast

Day 1

LiveJuice & More

- Green Live Juice and wheatgrass all day
- Drink a gallon of distilled water or ½ of your body weight in ounces
- Fresh squeezed lemon, 16oz. water and a dropperful *CayennePower* (or to taste) 3 times a day, hot or cold
- Garlic – juice 1 clove, 3 times a day
- Hydrotherapy (Ch. 12)
- Skin Brushing (Ch. 12)
- Exercise
- Fresh air and sunlight

Herbal Supplements

- *PowerGrab* 7-10 capsules 5 times a day/ *PowerGrab* Powder 1 tsp to 1 tbl 5 times a day
- *PowerFood*, 3 or more capsules 3 times a day
- *DetoxPower Tea*, 3 cups a day
- *LiverPower*, 1 dropperful 3 times day
- *PowerPoop* – double up

Weeks 2 & 4 • PowerHouse Fast

Day 2

LiveJuice & More

- Green Live Juice and wheatgrass all day
- Drink a gallon of distilled water or ½ of your body weight in ounces
- Fresh squeezed lemon, 16oz. water and a dropperful *CayennePower* (or to taste) 3 times a day, hot or cold
- Garlic – juice 1 clove, 3 times a day
- Hydrotherapy (Ch. 12)
- Skin Brushing (Ch. 12)
- Exercise
- Fresh air and sunlight

Herbal Supplements

- *PowerGrab* 7-10 capsules 5 times a day/ *PowerGrab* Powder 1 tsp to 1 tbl 5 times a day
- *PowerFood*, 3 or more capsules 3 times a day
- *DetoxPower Tea*, 3 cups a day
- *LiverPower*, 1 dropperful 3 times day
- *PowerPoop*, double-up

Weeks 2 & 4 • PowerHouse Fast

Day 3

LiveJuice & More

- Green Live Juice and wheatgrass all day
- Drink a gallon of distilled water or ½ of your body weight in ounces
- Fresh squeezed lemon, 16oz. water and a dropperful *CayennePower* (or to taste) 3 times a day, hot or cold
- Garlic – juice 1 clove, 3 times a day
- Hydrotherapy (Ch. 12)
- Skin Brushing (Ch. 12)
- Exercise
- Fresh air and sunlight

Herbal Supplements

- *PowerGrab* 7-10 capsules 5 times a day/ *PowerGrab* Powder 1 tsp to 1 tbl 5 times a day
- *PowerFood*, 3 or more capsules 3 times a day
- *DetoxPower Tea*, 3 cups a day
- *LiverPower*, 1 dropperful 3 times day
- *PowerPoop* double-up

Weeks 2 & 4 • PowerHouse Fast

Day 4

LiveJuice & More

- Green Live Juice and wheatgrass all day
- Drink a gallon of distilled water or ½ of your body weight in ounces
- Fresh squeezed lemon, 16oz. water and a dropperful *CayennePower* (or to taste) 3 times a day, hot or cold
- Garlic – juice 1 clove, 3 times a day
- Hydrotherapy (Ch. 12)
- Skin Brushing (Ch. 12)
- Exercise
- Fresh air and sunlight

Herbal Supplements

- *PowerGrab* 7-10 capsules 5 times a day/ *PowerGrab* Powder 1 tsp to 1 tbl 5 times a day
- *PowerFood*, 3 or more capsules 3 times a day
- *DetoxPower Tea*, 3 cups a day
- *LiverPower*, 1 dropperful 3 times day
- *PowerPoop* double-up

Weeks 2 & 4 • PowerHouse Fast

Day 5

LiveJuice & More

- Green Live Juice and wheatgrass all day
- Drink a gallon of distilled water or ½ of your body weight in ounces
- Fresh squeezed lemon, 16oz. water and a dropperful *CayennePower* (or to taste) 3 times a day, hot or cold
- Garlic – juice 1 clove, 3 times a day
- Hydrotherapy (Ch. 12)
- Skin Brushing (Ch. 12)
- Exercise
- Fresh air and sunlight

Herbal Supplements

- *PowerGrab* 7-10 capsules 5 times a day/ *PowerGrab* Powder 1 tsp to 1 tbl 5 times a day
- *PowerFood*, 3 or more capsules 3 times a day
- *DetoxPower Tea*, 3 cups a day
- *LiverPower*, 1 dropperful 3 times day
- *PowerPoop* double-up

Weeks 2 & 4 • PowerHouse Fast

Day 6

LiveJuice & More

- Green Live Juice and wheatgrass till 2pm
- Drink a gallon of distilled water or ½ of your body weight in ounces
- Fresh squeezed lemon, 16oz. water and a dropperful *CayennePower* (or to taste) 3 times a day, hot or cold
- Consume raw garlic in your juices today at least 10 cloves, this will help in assisting the liver for the liver flush tonight
- Hydrotherapy (Ch. 12)
- Skin Brushing (Ch. 12)
- Exercise
- Fresh air and sunlight

Herbal Supplements

- *PowerFood*, 3 or more capsules 3 times a day
- *DetoxPower Tea*, 3 cups a day
- *LiverPower*, 1 dropperful 3 times day
- PowerHouse Liver Flush (Ch. 13)

Weeks 2 & 4 • PowerHouse Fast

Day 7

LiveJuice & More

- Day of rest, you will not take any herbal supplements
- Live Green Juice and wheatgrass all day
- Drink a gallon of distilled water or ½ of your body weight in ounces
- Colonics or high enema (Ch. 12)

The last 7 days of this 30 day cleanse, add in BloodCleansing Power Tincture for 3 times a day and use this for 6 days on and 1 day off, for a total of 3 weeks. Continue after the fasting is over.

CHAPTER 17

LIFE AFTER FASTING

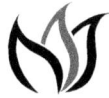

You're DONE! Welcome to "The Road Less Traveled."

BACK TO SOLIDS.

Clap, Clap! Applaud! I hear the crowd screaming!!!

Having gotten this far is a great feeling, and many will envy you for the dedication and perseverance you have shown. This was not necessarily an easy journey to embark on, short or long.

This knowledge, that you now have of your control over your own health and the ability to design your new destiny, many never realize they have this. Doesn't it feel GREAT?

When you're going back into eating after a fast, you want to take it slow. Don't gorge or you will undo some of your hard work. Stay with items similar to what you were juicing, greens and other fresh fruit and vegetable, to gently reintroduce your digestive system to solid food. Imagine not being a runner, and suddenly running the 5K. What a reckless undertaking that would be! It takes practice and a built-up endurance. Well, your digestive system works the same way.

- Eat lightly
- Eat fruit, vegetables, grains, nuts and seeds
- Drink plenty of liquids
- Drink water
- Drink juice
- Chew slowly
- Chew your food completely so your stomach is ready for it

Also, don't drink ANY liquids with your meals. Wonder why this advice? The answer is that our stomach works better when filled with a combination of just air, food, and its own gastric juices. Drinking liquids while eating, ultimately dilutes the acids that our stomach produces.

After a cleansing fast like this, you will become more aware of how food works with you and of your body's functions.

Welcome Back to Wholesome Foods

When I first got into this type of healing, I was learning how this all worked and how powerful the properties of fruits and vegetables were. I became vegetarian plus wheat/gluten free and dairy free, as I was allergic to those items. I thought that was the way to go, and believed it would help my body the best way I possibly could.

I stayed vegetarian for 2 years on this journey, but eventually my energy was getting increasingly lower and lower, and my weight was getting out of control. Someone suggested to me that I add shredded chicken to my salad, and the very next morning I dropped 7 pounds. No kidding! The next day after adding meat, instead of experiencing the typical drop in energy around noon, my energy level was incredibly high. Just one more lesson learned along my journey.

I find this worth repeating from my story,

My husband had a good analogy for this: Humans, like other meat-eating animals in the animal kingdom, have eye-teeth in addition to their flat molars. Animals that eat grass have flat teeth. If we have pointed teeth, it must be that we are designed to eat meat. It made sense! That is what led me to Sally Fallon's book, *Nourishing Traditions.* It is a worthwhile buy at:
 www.newtrendspublishing.com/SallyFallon/

Along the way, among the many classes I was taking, I landed in a class about eating wholesome foods, meats, and raw milk. When people in that group talked about raw milk, their eyes would just LIGHT up; they had this gaze in their eyes! I couldn't understand it. So I visited an organic milk farm and actually got the courage to try raw milk.

The first thing I noticed was the taste. It is delicious! I don't know how they can even call that stuff in the store "milk." There is no comparison! Now I have that gaze too. When milk is processed, the taste gets killed from the heat, and so do all the valuable nutrients. After I started drinking raw milk, my nails were incredibly strong, a benefit I noticed almost immediately. (But I have also noticed that I have to keep everything in moderation. I did start drinking too much of it, and then I got all gunked up in my nose and lungs.)

Once again, I learned something new, and I'm glad I did!

So from my findings through this natural healing process, I do believe it is very helpful to be on a vegetarian diet in the beginning to facilitate the healing. Then, once you are healed, return to a full array of wholesome foods!

For a great source about wholesome foods, visit: www.westonaprice.org

Chapter 18

Testimonials

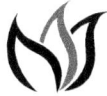

I was diagnosed with MS in December 2006. My neurologist said it was most likely the Primary Progressive type, as I did not seem to have any distinct remissions. Like most people, it was indescribably devastating to get this news and think my life and all my dreams were over. I won't go into detail about it here, but suffice it to say that I took it as hard as anybody could and that was the case for more than a year after the diagnosis. I lost most of my friends who could no longer listen to all my talk of doom-and-gloom. Even so, at my initial diagnosis I began doing research and quickly saw the conventional treatments helped very little, if at all. I was determined —and still am—not to have MS, and upon doing searches found a number of stories of people who healed MS and decided I would be one of them. About 9 months into my diagnosis I came across Gina Kopera's story. She was just beginning to launch Gina's Corner at that time. She told me about the cayenne tincture and even told me how to make it, but I preferred to purchase hers—which I did. Sure enough, it helped my bladder issues tremendously. Instead of having tremendous urinary urgency feelings and urinating tiny amounts up to 20 or more times a day (no exaggeration), with the tincture I began urinating only about 8 to 10 times per day and in larger volume. I have been using Gina's cayenne tincture on-and-off since that time. I use it whenever I feel my bladder/urination issues starting to act up again—and sure enough, it helps each time. I did try a cayenne tincture that I

purchased at a local healthfood store and at one point—and it did absolutely nothing for me. Luckily, they took it back and I have stuck with Gina's formula. I highly recommend this to anyone with frequent urination issues.

Moreover, around the time I first met Gina, she introduced me to the protocol that she used to conquer MS. She was extremely kind, positive, and supportive in her encouragement of my healing. I tried to do her protocol at that time (around the fall of 2007) but found I was unable to do the fasting part or the mucous-less diet. I would go a couple of days on the protocol, but then would continually give in to my food cravings. For the next year or so after that, I stopped trying Gina's protocol and went many other routes, including Low Dose Naltrexone (LDN), the Best Bet Diet (BBD) strictly for 4 months, having all the metals in my mouth removed, seeing three alternative practitioners, and trying numerous supplements. I believe these things probably helped me from having a major downward slide, but I did not see any improvement (except in the bladder issues). So a couple of months ago (January 2009), I decided to return to Gina's protocol. Since then I have done better with sticking with the juice fasting and the use of the intestinal cleansing herbs then I did the first time around. What's most remarkable though is that for the first time I am having new improvements—specifically my energy level is much higher and I have had significant reductions in numbness and stiffness of the extremities. I hardly have those symptoms at all, and it such a relief not to have that "hug" feeling around my lower right leg. Overall I just feel more like me again. (Improvements like these are not supposed to happen with Primary Progressive MS—according to my doctors anyway). I am so excited about these improvements and feel that for the first time in over 2 years I have some real hope of conquering MS, as Gina did. I am still struggling with staying on the juice fast but I am determined to do so, as I have some real hope now thanks to Gina. I have made, as Gina calls it, "conscious contact" with healing and knowing this is working. I owe an unbelievable debt of gratitude to Gina. I feel like I am getting my life back.

~ Andrea W.

_____

Hi Gina,

Just wanted to tell you how pleased I am with your products. I am very impressed with how quick my order was processed and shipped. I absolutely love the cayenne tincture as well as the Eye Formula. I've only used the Eye Formula once and immediately felt a "super clean" feeling that I haven't felt in over two years.

I can't thank you enough for being my mentor in this healing journey. Bless you for all you've been through and sharing what you have learned.

Your purpose in life is definitely being fulfilled to the fullest!

~ Carlin

———————————————

Dear Gina,

Xtreme Testimonial!

I am delighted to share with you my success in a newfound skin crème. At the age of 78 I have spent many years and much expense trying to find cosmetics that would help retard the onset of "old age" and been using top-of-the-line make-ups, thinking this had to be the answer. [Gina's product] PuraXtreme Crème has been the ultimate success. The moisturizer gives my face a marvelous anointing and after applying my foundation, leaves my face with a subtle shine or glow making me to feel radiant.

Thank you PuraXtreme Crème!

~ Rita, Arizona

———————————————

Hey Gina —

Regarding to the EnzymePower...

Not only do I not have heartburn anymore, BUT I CAN ALSO NOW DRINK ORANGE JUICE AGAIN!!

I have not been able to drink OJ for at least 3 years. It would stir up all the stomach acid until I felt my chest would explode with heartburn. I drank a 16oz OJ this morning, and I feel great!! I continue to be impressed!

~ Carla Lyons

———————————————

I have been to Gina's website. She is truly an inspiration. I would recommend checking out her site. She is an amazing woman with tremendous strength and determination to live the best possible quality of life in spite of her illness. And she has done some amazing things in regards to her illness. Just wanted to let everyone know and to support Gina!

Blessings,

Renee

———————————————

Dear Gina:

I just finished reading your website and just wanted to thank you for it. I was diagnosed with MS in 1995 and know what you went thru. Again I don't want to bother you or anything but just say thank you for being you.

~ Chuck

———————————————

Hi Gina,

I really want to thank you for all this coaching you are doing and taking your time and experience to help me. It is very, very kind of you, and I really appreciate it.

~ Anonymous

———————————————

Gina,

Today I finally took the time to completely review your site. You are to be commended for being persistent and resolving your issues. Your son's as well. More importantly, you are to be commended for taking the time out of your day to help others 'see the light'. I have been on a mission, though admittedly, more vigorously sometimes than others since I watched the movie "Lorenzo's Oil". It is a very impressive story of how a Mom and Dad had to go make their own discoveries. This is what you have done, and I am endeavoring to accomplish.

Thanks again! Michael

————————————

Dear Gina,

Distilled water:

Just wanted to tell you how well your recommendation to drink distilled water worked!!!! I had gone in for my annual exam and the doctor said there were traces of blood and crystals in my urine — indicating the start of kidney stones. Over 2 or 3 weeks I was checked 2 more times with the same result and sent to an urologist. I started drinking the distilled water and by the time I got to the urologist he couldn't figure out why I was there! There were no traces of blood or crystals and had to even double check the test results that were sent to his office. He wanted to know what I was doing because it was obviously working and he couldn't believe it was something so simple!

Lotion:

Your lotion is amazing!!! My skin was so dry with eczema and flaking like crazy. Your lotion took all the dryness away, helps my makeup go on better and actually makes me actually look younger! I've also used it on my son's hands — the eczema on his hands was so bad they would bleed and the lotion cleared it up within 2 days. I even gave a bottle to my babysitter's sister for her baby's eczema.

Cayenne:

Everything you have told me to do with the cayenne tincture has worked!!! A drop on my tongue cleared up a headache, it kills a sore throat instantly, I even put it on my lip when it got infected from when I tripped and bit it!

Detox tea:

I have to tell you how much I love the DetoxPower Tea! I've noticed a difference immediately. My energy level is up, I feel better, and my potassium is finally in check — without medication!!!! The best part is — it tastes great! I'm buying some for my boyfriend...!

~ Julie, Chicago

————————————

Gina,

Fasted 14 days if you count the 3 days it took on soup, apples & juice to break it. Lungs have cleared up. Swelling in lower legs almost completely gone. I am very happy with the results.

Larry, Iowa

———————————————————

Gina,

After my 28 day's on the PowerHouse Fast I felt better 50-60% better after 2 to the 3rd week, my balance was back, more energy I can make it through the whole day.

I can walk better with more confidence of not falling. The most impressive part was during the 3rd week of the PowerHouse Fast, I didn't even realize this until afterwards, and I lifted my own leg into the shower on its own, where prior I had to physical lift my leg with my hands to get it into the tub. Weight loss was about 30-35lbs on the fast (which was great and I have held it off too!), I can climb up and downs stairs defiantly more confident and faster.

After the fast I continued with whole food diet, the main part is greens, staying away from sugar and dairy. I still can walk better and gearing up for the next fast to pump it up another notch.

Dan, Iowa

———————————————————

Gina-

February of 2009 I started to notice slight tumors in my head. It was constant and very annoying. I decided I had a pinched nerve and took myself to a chiropractor, he told me that it is more serious than a pinched nerve, possibly a tumor in my brain! He sent me to a local doctor who suggested going to a neurologist. He then ordered a MRI which came back normal as he suspected; he diagnosed me with benign tremors, he explained, " It is like old people that have the shakes."

The doctor wanted me to take medication. That was something I didn't want to do for the rest of my life, being only 32 with two young children, it would be a lengthy time on medication and a lot of money.

My next step was to call you and see what remedies you had for me to try. The first step was get to pooping, which I was already doing and taking Cayenne power 3 times a day and she added to that NervPower and a one week juice fast.

I first continued with my regular diet and I cut out pop and drank a gallon of distilled water each day.

Few weeks later, I did the PowerGrab fast for 5 days and continued with water, cayenne and doubled the dose of PowerPoop. Instantly my tremors reduced to 98% by the end of that fast. I feel wonderful. Calling Gina for advice was the best thing that I ever done!

Angie Kopera, Milton, Iowa

CHAPTER 19

HOW TO MAKE SOME OF THESE PRODUCTS

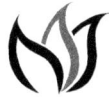

No, it doesn't take someone with a Ph.D. to be able to make these products in their own kitchen. It is amazing how easy it is to accomplish. We will start with a tincture, which really isn't time-consuming. Follow me and I will teach how easy this is for you to do.

Be sure you consult a health care professional if you are receiving any medical treatments or may have a serious health condition.

Grain Alcohol Tinctures

A tincture is an herbal preparation made by combining alcohol, distilled water or vinegar with dried or fresh herbs. The result can be consumed by mixing the tincture with tea, water, or juice, or by taking the tincture straight from a dropper or spoon.

One teaspoon taken up to three times daily should be the proper dosage for any herbal tincture. A tincture is the most effective method of using herbal medicines.

You can purchase dried and fresh herbs from your local natural food store, or find an online seller for dried herbs.

To begin, you will need pure grain alcohol. I like to use an 80-proof vodka, but you can go stronger. You could also substitute distilled water or apple cider vinegar, if you would like a non-alcoholic tincture.

> Note: Do not use rubbing alcohol or wood alcohol. To do so would be to create poison, not medicine. If using distilled water, this must be refrigerated.

What You Will Need

- Cheesecloth or (I prefer to use an old clean t-shirt that is thinner), then I can toss it after I am done.
- Mason jars, preferably an amber jar, brown paper and a dark storage area.
- Blender
- Coffee Grinder
- Glass bottles with a glass dropper

A health food store should have these items, or there are many companies online. The company that I started out using was www.essentialsupplies.com. They also sell all different kinds of amber bottles.

Folklore tells us to start preparing our tinctures on the day of the new moon and end on the following full moon. On this day, grind your herbs with a coffee grinder to get them finer as this will make your tincture stronger. Otherwise, put them into a blender.

If I am making cayenne tincture I fill a blender ¾ full with rinsed habaneras, then fill the rest of the way with vodka. Blend until chopped up.

Now put your herbs in a Mason jar. Seal it tightly so that it cannot leak or evaporate. Now put the tincture-to-be in a dark area, an unused closet or cabinet would be perfect. You may even want to cover it with a dark colored towel.

You will need to shake your tincture about the same time each day for about two weeks, or until the full moon. If you forget, don't worry, it will be okay. Just do your best to shake it every day.

When it is time to remove your tincture from storage, take out another mason jar, your brown paper, and cheesecloth or old clean t-shirt. Cut the cheesecloth to cover the mouth of the Mason jar. Screw the ring over the cloth, and then pour the liquid into the new jar. When you have poured all of the liquid into the new jar, take the straining cloth off the first jar.

Take a larger piece of cloth and pour the herbs into it. Now, squeeze the remaining liquid into your tincture. Seal your new tincture and wrap the Mason jar in brown paper to keep out light.

Never forget to also label your tincture to know exactly what you have and date the label. Store this in a cool dark place. Your tincture should be good for two years and possibly many years beyond that. I have read of people trying tinctures from 90 years ago and still being just as strong when made with alcohol.

Making Herbal Capsules

Easy to make and easy to take, herb capsules are virtually tasteless. They are also not as quickly absorbed into bloodstream as herbs taken in a tea or tincture, but they are handy, particularly for those on the go. By making your own capsules, you can create your own blend, perfectly suited to your needs.

Capsules come in different sizes, with "00" the standard adult size. One adult cap holds about one-half teaspoon of powdered herb, and two "00" caps are commonly considered a standard dose for an adult. You can use either non-gelatin, vegetarian caps, which are made from plant cellulose, or the more common gelatin caps.

When using an encapsulator that you buy from your health food store or online resource, then gelatin works far better; the vegan ones don't slide out of the encapsulator very easily. Note: When buying an encapsulator, make sure it has a tamper; this will give you more herb content in each capsule.

These are the different sizes that are generally offered:

You can encapsulate herbs by hand, in a small bowl, or with the help of an encapsulating machine. Make sure your hands are dry as you work, and consider combinations of powdered herbs for maximum effect.

Finding good quality herbs is very important to the effectiveness of your finished product and not all herbs are created equal, I will give you an example:

I was making a tincture with Red Clover Blossoms, that particular herb needs to be picked when the color of the blossom is a reddish purple to get full effectiveness. When I went locally to the stores that carried bulk herbs, the color of the Red Clover blossom was as brown as brown could be.

Suppliers of Quality Herbs

Mountain Rose Herbs – www.mountainroseherbs.com

Pacific Botanicals – www.pacificbotanicals.com

Starwest – www.starwest-botanicals.com

Blessed Herbs – www.blessedherbs.com

Amber dropper bottles, jars and The Capsule Machine you can find at: Mountain Rose www.mountainroseherbs.com

Amber Dropper Bottles, Jars

Essential supplies www.essentialsupplies.com

Make Your Own Lotion or Crème

Making your own lotion is very fun and very moisturizing!

It is so easy; if you can cook you can make this. It is a very good recipe. I suppose even if you don't cook you would be able to this — it is just a matter of melt and stir.

- 12 ounce of Distilled Water
- 1/2 ounce of E-Wax
- 1-1/4 ounce Stearic Acid
- 1 teaspoon of Vegetable Glycerin (natural preservative)
- 1 tablespoon of Vitamin E (natural preservative)
- 2 3/4 ounce of oils and butters
- 1/2 of a teaspoon of Xantham Gum (optional) this will help bind the ingredients together to ensure a batch so you don't have separation

Heat water, and oil or butters in two separate pots. Add e-wax and Stearic Acid to the oil or butter mixture.

When it reaches 110-120 degrees (do not go above 120, as it starts to destroy the great part of the oil) take from heat and mix the liquid and oil together. Use a stick blender to mix. Then put in a cool water bath (you fill the sink up with cold water and set the pot in the sink).

Blend with hand blender few more times.

Add your favorite essential oil. That's it!

Makes approximately 16 ounces.

Tricks to My Trade

- I never use a thermometer when I am using butters such as Shea Butter, Cocoa butter etc. I just watch until everything is melted then take it off the heat and mix with the distilled water.

- Distilled water is a must. Tap water will mold too fast.

- I always add some *CayennePower* to my lotion formula.

- I always make the distilled water part into a tea, using whatever herb would be soothing and helpful to your skin. (Calendula is a good one). You just need to experiment with the herb of your choice.

- Best preservatives in your lotion or crème are Vitamin E and vegetable glycerin. Add them to every batch. It will last much longer.

- Must refrigerate this crème or lotion to get a longer lifespan out of it. A small amount can be left out for convenience.

- Making a thicker crème add the harder butters, such as Cocoa butter, Shea butter, really anything that ends in butter. Beeswax is another good one. This will make a thicker cream, but also will make it oilier, which is great, for those with very dry skin. Use a lighter oil to make a lighter lotion or crème, with a not as oily feeling to the skin. Add oils such as coconut oil, avocado oil, olive oil, almond oil etc. There are a wide variety of choices you can make. Just experiment

- If you find the lotion is too thin, you might have to make a new batch with mainly butters to it. Then combine the two batches together to really thicken it up. Use a handheld blender to mix thoroughly.

I Personally Use

Cocoa butter, Mango butter, Shea butter, Almond oil, Castor oil, Wheat Germ oil, Vegetable Glycerin and Vitamin E oil are my favorites to use. Once you try this you will never want to go back. I do sell a crème formula called PuraXtreme Crème and, trust me, it will not clog pores. You ask why? This is all natural food for the skin. It will absorb through the layers not lie on them. Of course, I add a dropperful of *CayennePower* to each batch, the spice of life.

CHAPTER 20

THANK YOU LETTER

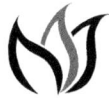

Whoosh, done! Thank you, God! It was not so terrible after all.

I merely wanted to give all my readers a note of thanks for reading my book.

This information is certainly thinking outside of the box. Once the method is applied, and you have had a conscious experience with this sort of healing you may wonder why you did not do it a long time ago.

My deepest hope is that it will help you, someone you love, or even someone you do not know at all!

I can't predict the future – no one can. But with the results I've seen and experienced first-hand in the present, I'll take the present.

"Yesterday is history. Tomorrow's a mystery. Today is a gift."

Thank you for your continued support!

Sincerely,

Gina Kopera, M.H.

APPENDIX

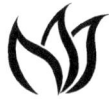

APPENDIX A

GINA'S CORNER PRODUCTS

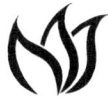

A man too busy to take care of his health is like a mechanic too busy to take care of his tools. That famous Spanish proverb still rings true today.

Establishing and maintaining good health greatly enhances the quality and longevity of your life!

What is the problem most people face? Poor health. The average person only reacts to health problems as they occur rather than adopting a consistent lifestyle that prevents easily preventable and debilitating illnesses from occurring in the first place. Good health also means *being proactive* - it doesn't just happen.

Healthy people work at it.

What Tools Are Available?

For centuries, herbs have been successfully used medicinal purposes. The naturally occurring healing properties help your body maintain proper function and balance and restore your body's vigor and vitality.

That's the good news. The bad news is...

The bad news is not all herbs are created equal. ***Most herbal companies sell cheap, poor-quality herbal mixes in pretty packaging.***

While competitors mark-up their products to cover expensive labels and packaging, Gina's Corner products are formulated with the highest quality and most effective herbs available for the lowest price anywhere!

An important fact you need to know is that every product contains the highest 2:1 ratio allowed by law! Our exclusive formulas contain rich, effective herbs. There are no cheap fillers and unlike most herbal products, none of Gina's Corner tincture formulas taste of alcohol!

Your Satisfaction Guarantee

Every product and every service available from this book is delivered to you with a 100% satisfaction guarantee at **www.ginascorner.com.**

PowerPoop

This is the very first place to start.

The retention and absorption of this toxic waste often results in unnecessary illnesses and disease that began as hard-to-diagnose symptoms masking the true problem.

The first step in anyone's health program should be stimulating, cleansing and toning all of the elimination organs. The bowel is the best place to begin and the PowerPoop Intestinal Formula is just the right combination of organic herbs to achieve this objective.

There is only one thing I am interested in, and that is RESULTS!

PowerGrab

This formula will also remove over 3,000 known drug residues. Its natural mucilaginous properties softens old, hardened fecal matter for easy removal and makes it an excellent remedy for any inflammation in the stomach and intestines.

EnzymePower

Restore your body's natural enzymes!

EnzymePower will aid in breaking down your food and will alleviate that full and bloated feeling.

Also stops burping, belching, heartburn, and acid indigestion!

DetoxPower Tea

PowerDetox Tea formulation designed to assist in flushing your skin, blood, liver and kidneys, leaving body systems feeling healthy.

Jr.Poop

Severe, untreated chronic constipation, even in our little ones, can lead to physical problems with the digestive tract and the body's metabolic systems and mental issues such as hyperactivity and ADD. Constipation is very common in children. Children who are constipated tend to have hard or painful stools or no bowel movement for four days or more. Smaller sized capsules for the younger ones to swallow.

Little Ones Do-Do

Untreated chronic constipation can lead to physical problems with the digestive tract and the body's metabolic systems, which accompanies many-sleepless nights for all!

Nasal Snuff

This potent blend of spicy snuff will instantly alleviate sinus congestion and pressure, while ridding you of the worst sinus headaches.

The Nasal Snuff formula performs a double duty. **It blows through the blockage of a stuffy nose and can stop a runny nose.**

PowerFood

PowerFood supplements assist in strengthening, toning, and stimulating your whole body.

The zero-fat formula will give you the quick, sustainable energy that your body needs, without slowing you down later.

This exclusive PowerFood alkalizing formula should be the foundation of any health program you are practicing.

PowerFood for Animals

This perfectly balanced blend, and specifically formulated to supply your pet with protein and essential amino acids for better muscle development and overall performance.

Pets need protein in order to grow and stay strong and it's the whole-food ingredients that your pet will gobble up.

HeatingPower Oil

Are you looking for a miracle in a bottle? Look no further, "Gina's Corner" has just what you need!

Our specially formulated to handle so many conditions; you will be surprised at how well it works and how versatile it is!

This is the perfect product to turn to when you bruise, bang, or when you have sprained a joint. **It literally turns two weeks of healing time into two days!**

PowerPuberty

Don't let the title fool you; PowerPuberty is perfect for all ages and genders!

You've tried coping. Now come, experience the other side of life, for a change. Nature's perfect blend of herbs to balance your hormones, stabilize mood swings plus powerful nutrients of all alkaline ingredients.

PowerBlood Cleanser

The bloodstream is your River of Life, so keep it clean!

This herbal blood re-builder is made up of cleansers and astringents which aid in removing cholesterol, purification, killing infections, blood cleansing, and in build¬ing elasticity and strength in the walls of the veins and arteries. Helps promote a healthy, clean bloodstream.

BrainPower Formula

Our brains are behind everything we do in life. Without us even having to think about it, they help us do everything from balancing our checkbook to buttoning our shirt in the morning.

It's imperative that we keep our brain in great working condition.

One of the most efficient ways to improve the function of your brain is to increase blood circulation. BrainPower Formula will boost your memory, improve circulation and has very effective anti-aging benefits.

CayennePower

Cayenne – *capsicum annum* – is considered by many to be the strongest stimulants known.

Internally use as a relaxant to the stomach and colon and as a healer for ulcers. It stimulates the stomach but is not irritating.

Cayenne stimulates the blood and the heart, increasing and strengthening the pulse. Use for colds, sinus, respiratory ailments, indigestion, hangover, diabetes, cramps, circulation problems, asthma, rheumatism, kidneys, high blood pressure, fungus underneath the nails and stops bleeding immediately on a open cut.

No one should be without this bottle!

When in doubt, just give it a try!

Your satisfaction is 100% guaranteed!

EchinaceaPower Formula

Supercharges your immune system, combats diseases and infections.

EchinaceaPower will help build and boost the immune system to strengthen and tone your body so that you can fight off these different infections.

EyePower Formula

This eyewash cleanses and strengthens the eyes. It contains cayenne, don't let that scare you, this formula wouldn't have the power-charge that it does without it. This eyewash cleanses and strengthens the eyes. It increases blood circulation to the eyes and assist in removing toxic waste in and around the eyes. It also can assist in reversing eye diseases and destroying bacterial infections.

KidneyPower

This tincture is both a diuretic (increases the flow of urine) and disinfectant (destroys urinary tract infections) great for the kidneys, bladder, and urinary system. It will assist in soften and breaking up inorganic salts and minerals that have collected in those areas.

LiverPower

The liver is one of the most important organs, so keep it strong and healthy. When the liver is working properly, the digestive system works better and the skin glows. **Your liver is a blood-cleaning filter.** It protects you by cleaning toxic chemicals and poisons from food, water, air and the environment from your blood.

LobeliaPower

LobeliaPower has a therapeutic action as an anti-spasmodic, a bronchial dilator, and an expectorant. As an anti-spasmodic, it is second to none! It will relax the entire body and its organs. It is the greatest herb for lungs problems, as well!

RedRasberry

Red Raspberry Leaves support the reproductive system, especially during pregnancy.

Assists in balancing out hormones in children going through puberty and in women suffering PMS.

WomanPower

Did you know you can take more control over your monthly menstruation, menopause, or PMS? You can! WomanPower is an amazing combination of finest-quality herbs that aid in building your system to alleviate these common menstruation problems.

Champion Juicer

Your Champion 2000+ Juicer is designed to produce the highest possible quality of juices and foods. It's a difference you can see in the color of the juice: darker, richer colors contain more of the pigments - and nutrients - you desire, while the extracted pulp is pale in color. And rest assured, it's a difference you can taste. Champion juices will likely be richer, sweeter and more full-bodied than any juice you've tasted before.

PuraXtreme Anti-Aging Crème

PuraXtreme will not only bring relief to the skin it will also, assist in healing and repairing. This is a winning combination of oils, butters and herbs that will strengthen and nourish your skin. It will have lasting benefits, unlike most lotions. It can help bring back a youthful appearance. Fresh is always best, and you will love it.

Personalized Coaching

Curious about how to heal your body with herbs, but not quite sure where to start? You have come to the right place!

As a master herbalist, I have the education, skills and experience to **help you**

enjoy optimal health and energy faster than you ever thought possible.

What You Will Receive

Reserve a private coaching session from one of the options below and you will receive personalized, expert advice for resolving:

- Pain
- Blood pressure
- Indigestion
- Sinus pressure
- Headaches
- Constipation
- Heartburn
- Menstruation problems
- Cholesterol

Plus extraordinary solutions for any other health challenges!

The benefits of natural healing, in most cases, far outweigh traditional prescription medication. Give your body and well-being the opportunity to **experience the benefits of our exclusive herbal formulas** at www.ginascorner.com Get a no obligation, free evaluation at info@ginascorner.com.

The personalized assessment, one-on-one attention, and care you will receive can very quickly give you a whole new outlook on life.

Your Privacy Guarantee

Your complete privacy is 100% assured. Additionally, no questions are just "stock answers," recycled from person to person. As a valued client, you will receive a very personalized response specific to your questions and health needs.

Coaching Service Options

Priority Response Coaching

This service is ideal if you would like priority response to a question specific to your needs within 24 hours of submission:

- Not sure what an herbal product or ingredient is used for?

- Can a certain product be used in conjunction with other herbs?

- Which product is the best match for my situation?

Select this service and receive a detailed, personalized response to your question. After you have completed your order, you may submit your questions from our contact page OR simply respond to the email we send you.

Cleansing Coaching Package

This package is ideal to get started with a complete herbal program and includes the answers specific to your needs so you receive the exact products that will benefit you most.

You'll receive instructional assistance to experience a shorter cleansing process. Whether you follow a 5 to 10 day fasting through the Mucous-Free protocol or through the JuicePower protocol, this program will meet your needs. **I guarantee you will begin feeling better than ever!**

Complete support for the JuiceHouse Fasting Program or the Mucous-Free Diet. Package Includes:

Two weeks of daily coaching thru phone or email • 165 page eBook instant download• PowerPoop Intestinal Formula • PowerGrab Intestinal Formulae • DetoxPower Tea • PowerFood• LiverPower • CayennePower • KidneyPower • BloodCleansing Tincture • EchinaceaPower • **Over $180 in herbal products!**

PowerHouse Coaching Package

Complete support for the PowerHouse Fasting Program. Package includes:

One month of daily coaching thru phone or email• 165 page eBook instant download• 2-PowerPoop Intestinal Formula • 4-PowerGrab Intestinal Formulae • DetoxPower Tea • PowerFood• LiverPower • CayennePower • KidneyPower • BloodCleansing Tincture • EchinaceaPower • **Over $290 in herbal products!**

My Medical Records

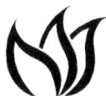

THE NEBRASKA MEDICAL CENTER
CLARKSON HOSPITAL - UNIVERSITY HOSPITAL
Nebraska Medical Center
Omaha NE. 6B198
KOPERA. GINA M.
MRN: 00765776 SEX: F
DOB: 3Jun68
Test Date/Time: 1998-04-21:00:00
Entry/Dictating: BASHIR, RIFAAT
Report Name: History and Physical. Clinical

--NURSING HISTORY --

EVALUATION FOR MULTIPLE SCLEROSIS. 2ND OPINION

REASON FOR VISIT: MULTIPLE SCLEROSIS

--NURSING VITAL SIGNS --

WEIGHT KG 164.1 LB (74.6 KG)

BLOOD PRESSURE 124/64 RIGHT ARM SITTING

PULSE RATE 76 Reg Sit

--HISTORY OF PRESENT ILLNESS--

This is a 29 year old, right-handed, white female who is here for a second opinion on the diagnosis of multiple sclerosis given to her in May 1997. The diagnosis was made after the patient woke up one day in March 1997 with tingling and numbness in the left hand, arm, and leg. This tingling has been present since that time. Of note is that the thumb and index finger bothered her the most. Initially she was told that she had carpal tunnel syndrome. Subsequently she developed left lower extremity and left face tingling. Her diagnosis was changed to possible MS. An MRI scan of the cervical spine as well as CSF studies, were consistent with the diagnosis of MS. However, we don't know the actual results of the CSF exam, and the patient does not know either. The MRI showed some cervical spinal cord lesions as well as one periventricular lesion on the head MRI and another subcortical lesion. The patient reports having at that time a positive Lhermitte's sign. When she bent her neck, she would experience electrical-like tingling going down to her legs, especially the right leg. Most of the patient's symptoms at that time and still to date come when she is tired or gets exposed to heat. Otherwise, she has been feeling well since March 1997. The patient says today that she has not experienced any other episodes of weakness, numbness, tingling, loss of vision, blurred vision, or other neurological symptoms. The patient does not have any difficulty with bowel control. She does not have any problem with swallowing or visual changes. She does wear contact lenses, and she does have some refractive error which is getting worse. She is here today for a second opinion about the diagnosis of multiple sclerosis.

--ALLERGIES--

No known medical allergies.

--MEDICATIONS--

She is on Triphasil which is a birth control pill, she is on no other medications.

--PAST MEDICAL HISTORY--

Patient had a C-section times one and had genital herpes which has been dormant for many years. She has a history of having been knocked unconscious at age five years, the unconsciousness lasted from morning to night that day. She woke up after that and had no further problems.

--SOCIAL HISTORY--

She does smoke one pack per day, and she is a social drinker. She is married, and is employed. In particular, she does manicures which requires fine finger movement, the tingling affects her fine motor dexterity and interferes with her work.

--FAMILY HISTORY--

She had a paternal grandmother who had MS, and she has other family members with diabetes and cancer on both sides of her family.

--REVIEW OF SYSTEMS--

HEAD AND NECK: No visual problems. No Lhermitte's sign at the present time. No vertigo. No facial numbness.

RESPIRATORY: No dyspnea, cough, or wheezing.

CARDIOVASCULAR: No shortness of breath, orthopnea, leg swelling, palpitations, or chest pain.

GASTROINTESTINAL: No constipation. No sphincteric problems. No abdominal pain.

GENITOURINARY: No bladder dysfunction. No sphincteric abnormalities. No urgency. No retention of urine.

MUSCULOSKELETAL: Apart from the tingling and

---

numbness that she still has on the left side, the patient has no other abnormalities or complaints. However, she complains of generalized fatigue which she experiences with exposure to heat.

--GENERAL--

The patient is comfortable and in no acute distress. She is very pleasant.

--HEAD AND NECK--

Head: The face is symmetrical.

Eyes: Sclerae are slightly congested. The patient is wearing contact lenses.

Neck: No lymph nodes. No carotid bruits. No neck stiffness.

--LUNGS--

Clear to auscultation. No wheezing.

--HEART/CARDIOVASCULAR--

Regular rhythm and rate. No S3 and no murmur.

--ABDOMEN--

Abdomen is soft. Bowel sounds are positive. No organomegaly.

--EXTREMITIES--

There is no cyanosis or edema. The capillary refill is about one second.

--NEUROLOGIC--

Cranial nerve II: Visual acuity is 20/30 bilaterally. Visual fields are intact. and the optic disks are sharp bilaterally.

Cranial nerves III, IV, and VI: Extraocular muscles are intact. The pupils react equally to direct and consensual light constricting from 4.0 mm to 2.0 mm.

Facial sensation and muscles of mastication are normal. No facial asymmetry. She can close her eyes bilaterally quite tightly with mild asymmetry. Hearing is normal. Shoulder shrug is normal. Tongue is in the midline. and the uvula elevates symmetrically.

Motor Exam: Strength is 5/5 distally and proximally in the lower extremities. DTR's are symmetrical bilaterally being 2 in all muscle groups of biceps, triceps, brachioradialis, and at the knee and ankle. Plantar is downgoing bilaterally. Finger-to-nose is normal. Romberg sign is negative. Gait is completely normal. Lhermitte's sign is not present.

Sensory examination shows some abnormalities to temperature and touch on the left side of the body, especially on the left face and left hand. However, the left arm and leg are normal. On the trunk, the exam is inconsistent and sometimes showed inconsistent left trunk changes to touch. The vibration and the position senses are normal.

ASSESSMENT

Probable multiple sclerosis. We have reviewed her spinal and brain MRI, and there is definitely a lesion in the C-spine that is consistent with demyelination, and there are at least two lesions on brain MRI that are consistent with demyelination. However, despite the fact that the patient did have a clinical episode and there are some objective findings on the physical examination, it is still only one episode. For that reason, there is no dissemination in time yet, and so the patient has a diagnosis of probable multiple sclerosis. We will be following her over time. In case she develops another episode that is different from the one she is currently having, we will diagnose her as having definite multiple sclerosis and discuss treatment options at that time.

PLAN

We will see the patient in six months.

TEACHING PHYSICIAN PARTICIPATION

I personally interviewed, examined, and determined the key portions of this patient's medical service as follows:

HISTORY:

This is a 29 year old, right-handed, white female who is self-referred for a second opinion regarding the possibility of having multiple sclerosis. In early April 1997, Gina woke up one morning with tingling and numbness of her left hand. She is a beautician, and she noticed it initially in her index finger and thumb. Gradually, she noticed that this unusual sensation spread to her upper arm, trunk, and left lower extremity. She was seen by Dr. Harris Frankel on April 21, 1997, who documented a normal neurological examination except for some hypesthesia of the left arm, especially over the thenar eminence. He also noticed hypesthesia of the left trunk up to T7-8. The patient underwent an MRI of her cervical spine which showed a C4-5 signal abnormality. She underwent a spinal tap on April 22, 1997, that was reported as normal according to the notes. The patient subsequently developed Lhermitte's sign and was given a course of steroids. The patient improved gradually but remained with the area of hypesthesia over her left arm and chest. Since that time, the patient's Lhermitte's sign resolved gradually, but she continued to have a funny sensation in her left upper extremity like she has an extra layer of clothes over it. Of relevance is that the patient does not give a history of neck trauma, neck pain, or weakness. She has a history of genital herpes.

PHYSICAL EXAMINATION:

Vital signs are normal with a blood pressure of 124/64 mm Hg, pulse 76 per minute and regular, and weight 74.6 kg.

The patient is awake, alert, oriented, and retentive. Her language function is normal. Her recent and remote recall is normal. Cranial nerve examination including the visual system, extraocular motility, cranial nerve VII, cranial nerve VIII, and cranial nerves IX-XII are normal. She has good muscle bulk, power, and tone. Her reflexes are brisk but symmetrical in all four extremities. On sensory examination, the only abnormality we find is an area of hyposthesia including her left arm up to the shoulder and chest up to about T10. She also has some hypesthesia in her left lower extremity. Babinski sign is absent bilaterally. Coordination testing is performed adequately.

LABORATORY AND X-RAY DATA:

We reviewed the patient's MRI scan of the head, and it shows two tiny areas of signal abnormality. Her cervical spine MRI is more remarkable in that it shows an area of abnormal signal in the spinal cord at the C3-4 level. I reviewed the spinal fluid examination results, and they are normal.

ASSESSMENT:

Gina had a single bout of sensory abnormality involving her left arm, trunk, and left lower extremity with Lhermitte's sign that has improved but not resolved completely. I do not think we can make a diagnosis of multiple sclerosis on her based on this single attack. We explained to Gina that this could be a first episode of multiple sclerosis versus an attack of myelitis. She has gone a year without having any other new symptoms. At this point in time, we cannot make a diagnosis of definite multiple sclerosis on Gina.

PLAN:

Gina will come back and see us in about six months. She will call us earlier, and we will see her immediately should she have any other symptoms.

JINAN AL-OMAISHI, M.D.
SIGNED 5/19/98 7:23 AM

THE NEBRASKA MEDICAL CENTER
CLARKSON HOSPITAL - UNIVERSITY HOSPITAL
Nebraska Medical Center
Omaha NE. 68198
KOPERA. GINA M.
MRN: 00765776 SEX: F
DOB: 3Jun68
Test Date/Time: 1998-08-28:00:00
Entry/Dictating: BASHIR. RIFAAT
Report Name: Progress Note. Clinical

PROBLEM #Z PHONE CALL

SUBJECTIVE

Gina has been experiencing increased fatigue but is sleeping well during the night and is wondering if she can try
some medication for this. We will start Amantadine 100 mg
one b.i.d. She is to continue this for two to three weeks and
follow up on results of this medication.

> *SIGNED 9/8/98 5:30 PM, MARY FILIPI, F*
> *SIGNED 9/11/98 1:24 PM, RIFAAT BASHIR. M.D.*

THE NEBRASKA MEDICAL CENTER
CLARKSON HOSPITAL - UNIVERSITY HOSPITAL
Nebraska Medical Center
Omaha NE. 68198
KOPERA. GINA M.
MRN: 00765776 SEX: F
DOB: 3Jun68
Test Date/Time: 1999-01-22:00:00
Entry/Dictating: BASHIR, RIFAAT
Report Name: Progress Note. Clinical

-- NURSING HISTORY --

F/U MS AND WEAKNESS IN LEFT LEG.

REASON FOR VISIT: FOLLOWUP VISIT

--NURSING VITAL SIGNS --

WEIGHT KG 162.8 LB (74.0 KG)

BLOOD PRESSURE 122/70 RIGHT ARM SITTING

PULSE RATE 80 Reg Sit

TYMPANIC TEMPERATURE (F) 98.6

QUIET RESPIRATIONS 16

--MEDICATIONS ADMINISTERED IN CLINIC--

TUBERCULIN PURIFIED PROTEIN (SCLAVOTEST PPD MULTI PUNCTURE) INJECTION 0.1 U

PPD UPPER RIGHT ARM, CONTROL LOWER RIGHT ARM COME TO HAVE PPD READ MONDAY.

ADMINISTERED:1/22/1999 PROVIDERS:COFFEY. BASHIR

THE NEBRASKA MEDICAL CENTER
CLARKSON HOSPITAL - UNIVERSITY HOSPITAL
Nebraska Medical Center
Omaha NE. 68198
KOPERA. GINA M.
MRN: 00765776 SEX: F
DOB: 3Jun68
Test DatelTime: 1999-07-22:00:00
Result Status:
Entry/Dictating: AL-OMAISHI, JINAN
Report Name: Progress Note. Clinical
PROBLEM #Z TELEPHONE CALL

SUBJECTIVE:
Gina has called and states that she continues to have significant side effects on Avonex even at 1/2 dose. We will start her on 10 mg of oral prednisone with the shot in the morning after. If she continues to have side effects of a significant nature with this, we will consider changing agents.

MARY FILIPI, F
SIGNED 8/16/99 3:29 PM
JINAN AL-OMAISHI. M.D.

THE NEBRASKA MEDICAL CENTER
CLARKSON HOSPITAL - UNIVERSITY HOSPITAL
Nebraska Medical Center
Omaha NE. 68198
KOPERA, GINA M.
MRN: 00765776 SEX: F
DOB: 3Jun68
Test Date/Time: 1999-08-12:00:00
Entry/Dictating: MARKOPOULOU, EKATERINI
Report Name: Progress Note. Clinical

-- NURSING HISTORY --

PT HERE FOR FOLLOW UP VISIT REGARDING MULTIPLE
SCLEROSIS

REASON FOR VISIT: FOLLOWUP VISIT

--NURSING VITAL SIGNS --

WEIGHT KG 178.4 LB (81.1 KG)

BLOOD PRESSURE 126/66 LEFT ARM SITTING LARGE
CUFF

PULSE RATE 72 Reg Sit

* *

PROBLEM #2 MULTIPLE SCLEROSIS

SUBJECTIVE

Gina is a 31-year-old, right-handed, white female, presenting for followup of multiple sclerosis. She was last seen
January 22, 1999. She has since been started on Avonex 30
mcg 1M weekly and has had some significant side effects
from that. She is now on a partial dose and taking prednisone with each shot. This is working well. She did have

an episode of spasticity under the left arm and chest that lasted several hours. This was relieved by Motrin. Her muscles continued to be sore in that area for approximately four days. She identifies the discomfort as spasm-like. She has noted periodic occasional pain in her hands and arms but this goes away with no residual. She has had one episode of blurred vision in the left eye that lasted approximately 12 hours. Left arm and leg heaviness occurs with fatigue lasting approximately two to three hours only. She is up to the bathroom one time at night. She does experience urgency with urination but no signs or symptoms of urinary tract infection.

Gina does identify depression that has been occurring over the last several months. She denies any considerations of self harm but does notice that she cries considerably.

She has had some imbalance and walking problems that are sporadic in nature and lasting short periods of time. There is some concern about thinning of the hair on her head but she was reassured that this was more than likely not related to her disease process.

REVIEW OF SYSTEMS

No fevers or significant weight changes. She has had no chest pain, shortness of breath nor palpitations. She has not been incontinent of bladder or bowel.

Allergies: No known medical allergies.

Medications: Avonex 15 mg 1M weekly; Triphasil one po q.d.; prednisone 10 mg two weekly.

OBJECTIVE

Vital signs reveal blood pressure 126/66, pulse 72 and regular. and weight is 81.1 kg or 178.7 pounds. General health reveals Gina to be a well-developed female appearing her stated age and in no apparent acute distress. Head is normocephalic without lesions or masses noted. Neck is supple with full range of motion. She has no thyromegaly or lymphadenopathy present. Trachea is midline. Carotids are palpable at 2/4 without bruits. Lung fields are clear with good air movement throughout. Heart rate is regular without murmurs or rubs. Extremities are without edema.

NEUROLOGICAL EXAMINATION

COGNITIVE/LANGUAGE: Language pattern is normal without dysarthria. She is alert and oriented to time and place with good recent and remote recall. There are no cognitive deficits noted on examination.

CRANIAL NERVES:

I: Olfactory - Deferred.

II: Optic - Visual acuity is unchanged. Visual fields are intact.

III, IV and VI: Oculomotor, trochlear, and abducens - Pupils are equal and respond well to light. Funduscopic exam is unremarkable. Extraocular movements reveal an incomplete INO, particularly noticeable on left lateral movement.

V: Trigeminal - Sensation to light touch is intact over all three branches.

VII: Facial - Facial features are symmetrical with good muscle movement throughout.

VIII: Acoustic - Gross hearing is intact.

IX, X and XII: Glossopharyngeal, vagus, hypoglossal - Soft palate rises to the midline. Tongue is midline without deviation or fasciculation. Gag reflex is present.

XI: Accessory nerve - Shoulder shrug is strong and equal bilaterally.

MOTOR MUSCLE: Muscle groups are full without atrophy,

fasciculations, contractures, spasticity or rigidity. No prona-tor drift is present. Overall body strength is excellent at 5/5.

REFLEXES: Upper body reflexes are 2/4 bilaterally. Patellar reflexes are 3+/4 on the right, 3/4 on the left with ankle jerk at 3/4 bilaterally. Hoffmann and Babinski are absent.

SENSORY: There are no sensory changes noted. Pain, touch, and proprioception are intact. Romberg is absent.

CEREBELLAR: Coordination testing is excellent with fin-ger-to-nose, fine motor movement, and alternating move-ment. She is able to do heel-to-shin without difficulty.

GAIT: Gina demonstrates a narrow gait with good arm swing. She can walk on heels, toes, and tandem walk with-out difficulty.

ASSESSMENT

1) Multiple sclerosis-relapsing remitting

Overall, Gina is doing quite well with manageable side ef-fects with Avonex.

We will continue to give her partial doses. She has asked for medications for emergent depression and we will start her on Prozac 10 mg q.h.s. She has had no discrete flares since her last exam, and there has been some improvement of strength and reflexes since that time. We will continue her treatment plan with no changes but the addition of Prozac.

PLAN

1. Continue Avonex at partial dosing with monitoring lab work drawn today.

2. Initiate Prozac 10 mg q.h.s. with consideration to increase that as needed.

3. She is to return to clinic in three to four months and call us in the interim if any problems arise.

MARY FILIPI, F
SIGNED 9/8/99 11:35 AM
KATERINA MARKOPOULOU. M.D.

PROBLEM #2 MS

SUBJECTIVE

Gina is a 30-year-old right-handed white female presenting for follow-up of multiple sclerosis. She was last seen 4-21-98. At that time it was felt that she had probable multiple sclerosis but symptoms were not disseminated in time. Gina has now noticed the coming and going of symptoms with increased weakness in the left leg. This would give her dissemination in time for a diagnosis of multiple sclerosis. She has noted increased problems when she is tired or under stress. There is decreased sensation in the left leg with decrease in strength. She has an area described as a blank spot in the left thigh approximately 7-10 cm ovoid shaped since September or October. She has noticed an increased tremor in the hands bilaterally and stiffness in the left leg in the knee and below. She has had two unexplained falls on the same weekend in October. These falls occurred during a nonsymptomatic period. Severe headaches were present for two days in November with no vision changes. These have gone away and have not returned. Gina feels there has been increased memory problems also. There has been increased dyspnea in the morning when waking. These are short lived and are not related to any type of activity. She does not have any problems with exertional dyspnea. She currently has a head cold with some eye drainage.

Review of systems reveals no significant weight loss or fevers. She has had no chest pain, palpitations, exertional angina or dyspnea as previously reported. There has been no change in bowel or bladder habits.

Allergies: No known medical allergies.

Current medications: Amantidine and Depo-Provera.

Medical history is unchanged. She continues to smoke one pack per day.

OBJECTIVE

Vital signs: Blood pressure is 122/70, temperature is 98.6, pulse is 80, respirations are 16, weight is 74 kg.

General health - Gina is a well developed female appearing her stated age in no apparent acute distress. Head is normocephalic without lesions or masses noted. Neck is supple with full range of motion with no thyromegaly or lymphadenopathy present. Trachea is midline. Carotids are palpable at 2/4 without bruits. Lung fields are clear with good air movement throughout. Heart rate is regular without murmur or rubs. Extremities are without edema. Integument is intact.

Cognitive/language: Language pattern is normal with no dysarthrias. She is alert and oriented to time and place with good recent and remote recall. There are no gross cognitive deficits noted on exam.

Cranial nerves:

I. Olfactory - Deferred.

II. Optic - Visual acuity is unchanged. Visual fields are intact.

III, IV, VI - Oculomotor, trochlear and abducens: Pupils are equal and react well to light. Funduscopic exam is unremarkable Extraocular movements are intact without nystagmus.

V. Trigeminal - Sensation to light touch over ophthalmic, maxillary and mandibular areas is intact.

VII. Facial - Facial features are symmetrical with good muscle movement throughout.

VIII. Acoustic - Gross hearing intact.

IX, X, XII. Glossopharyngeal, vagus, hypoglossal - Soft palate rises to the midline. Tongue is midline without deviation or fasciculation. Gag reflex is present.

XI. Accessory nerve - Shoulder shrug is strong and equal bilaterally.

Motor/muscle: Muscle groups are full without atrophies, fasciculations, contractures, spasticity or rigidity. There is no pronator drift present. Upper body strength is excellent at 5/5. There is a slight decrease in the left hip flexors at 4+/5 and remaining muscle strength is 5/5 throughout.

Reflexes - Upper reflexes are normal at 2/4. Patellar reflexes are 3/4 on the right and 3+/4 on the left with heel cord at 2/4 bilaterally. Hoffman and Babinski's are absent.

Sensory - As reported previously there is a 7-10 cm ovoid patch on the left lower thigh with decreased sensation to pin prick. There are no other sensory levels present. Pain, touch and proprioception are intact. Romberg is absent.

Cerebellar - Coordination testing is excellent with finger to nose, fine motor movement, alternating movement. She is able to do heel to shin without difficulty.

Gait - Gina demonstrates a narrow gait with good arm swing. She can walk on her heels and toes and tandem walk without difficulty.

ASSESSMENT

Gina has shown dissemination in time with flareup of symptoms over the last month. We at this time feel it is appropriate to start treatment with beta interferon. This was discussed at great length with Gina and she concurs with this treatment plan. We will proceed with set up and initial testing related to Avonex therapy.

PLAN

1. TB test with control will be placed today. Initial lab work will be drawn.

2. We will start Avonex 30 meg 1M weekly. She is to return to the clinic after four to six doses if this is done. Further evaluation will be done at that time.

This dictation and assessment were done in conjunction with Dr. R. Bashir.

SIGNED 2/5/99 7:41 PM, MARY FILIPI. F
SIGNED 2/6/99 9:05 PM, RIFAAT BASHIR. M.D.

THE NEBRASKA MEDICAL CENTER
CLARKSON HOSPITAL - UNIVERSITY HOSPITAL
Nebraska Medical Center
Omaha NE. 68198
KOPERA. GINA M.
MRN: 00765776 SEX: F
DOB: 3Jun68
Test Date Time: 1999-10-21:00:00
Entry/Dictating: MARKOPOULOU, EKATERINI
Report Name: Progress Note. Clinical

--NURSING HISTORY --

PT. HERE FOR A FOLLOWUP VISIT REGARDING MULTIPLE SCLEROSIS.

REASON FOR VISIT: FOLLOWUP VISIT

--NURSING VITAL SIGNS--

WEIGHT KG 170.9 LB (77.7 KG)

BLOOD PRESSURE 108/70 LEFT ARM SITTING LARGE CUFF

PULSE RATE 80 Reg Sit

--CLINIC LABORATORY --

4:42 PM BLOOD GLUCOSE RANDOM 100

* *

PROBLEM #2 MULTIPLE SCLEROSIS

SUBJECTIVE

Gina is a 31 y/o right-handed white female presenting for
follow-up of multiple sclerosis and complaints of left eye
pain. She states it feels like a pulled muscle and does give
her considerable discomfort with lateral movement only.
She is questioning a blank spot in the left eye and does feel
there is a curtain-like effect present. It is light-sensitive.
The diplopia and discomfort in the eye occurred approximately two to three weeks ago with it progressing to pain
approximately two days ago. She has also noted numbness
in the left hand which was of brief duration two to three
days ago. She does have increased tingling and increased
dropping of things from that hand. Gina has recently started Avonex the end of June and is taking that with no problem. There has been no side-effects. She has had no other
type of symptom flare since that time.

Review of Systems: No fevers, significant weight change,
chest pain, shortness of breath, or palpitations. There has
been no change in her ability to chew, speak, or swallow.
She has noted no problems with bowel or bladder. She continues to work full-time. She tolerates the activity well.

ALLERGIES: None known.

Current Medications: Avonex 30 meg 1M weekly, Triphasil
one PO q day, and Aleve PO b.i.d. PRN pain.

OBJECTIVE

Vital signs - BP 108/70, pulse 80 and regular, wt. 77.7 kg or 171.3 pounds.

General - she is a well-developed, slender, female appearing her stated age and in no apparent acute distress.

HEENT - Normocephalic without lesions or masses noted.

Neck - supple with full range of motion with no thyromegaly or lymphadenopathy present. Trachea is midline. Carotid are palpable at 2/4 without bruits.

Lungs - clear with good air movement throughout.

Heart - regular without murmurs or rubs.

Extremities - without edema.

Neurologic -

Cognitive/Language - Language pattern is normal without dysarthria. She is alert and oriented to time and place with good recent and remote recall. There are no gross cognitive deficits noted on exam.

Cranial Nerves:

I: Olfactory - deferred.

II: Optic - Visual acuity is 20/40 OD, 20/70 OS. Visual fields appear to be intact, however, she does notice a central blurring in the left eye.

III, IV, & VI - Oculomotor, trochlear, and abducens: Left eye does demonstrate a mild inward drift. A horizontal diplopia is identified on left lateral movement. Extraocular movements appear to be intact with no nystagmus noted. Fundoscopic exam is unremarkable. PERRL, no Marcus-Gunn is present.

V: Trigeminal - Sensation to light touch is intact over all three branches.

VII: Facial - Facial features are symmetrical with good muscle movement throughout.

VIII: Acoustic - Gross hearing is intact.

IX, X, and XII: Glossal, pharyngeal, vagus, and hypoglossal - The soft palate rises to the midline. The tongue is midline without deviation or fasciculation. Gag reflex is present.

XI - Accessory - Shoulder shrug is strong and equal bilaterally.

Motor - Muscle groups are full without atrophy, fasciculations, contractures, spasticity or rigidity. There is no pronator drift noted. Overall body shoulder strength is good at 5/5.

Reflexes: Upper body reflexes are normal at 1-2/4, they are brisk on the lower extremities at 3/4 bilaterally. Hoffman and Babinski are absent.

Sensory - there are no sensory changes noted. Pain, touch, and proprioception are intact. Romberg is absent.

Cerebellar - coordination testing is excellent, with finger-to-nose, fine motor movement and alternating movement. She is able to do heel-to-shin with no signs of ataxia.

Gait - She demonstrates a narrow gait with good arm swing. She can walk on heel-to-toe and tandem walk without difficulty.

ASSESSMENT

1) Relapsing, remitting multiple sclerosis. EDSS 1.5.

2) Optic neuritis related to multiple sclerosis, accompanied by eye pain.

PLAN

A five-day steroid burst will be initiated and followed by an oral steroid taper. She is to continue the Avonex per standard protocol. She is to return to clinic in approximately three or four weeks, to follow-up in the interim if any problems arise.

Initial IV treatment will be started in the treatment center with the remainder done in the home by Quarum Health Care.

This dictation and assessment were done in conjunction with Dr. Markopoulou.

SIGNED 10/29/99 5:39 PM
MARY FILIPI. F
SIGNED 11/15/99 5:24 PM
KATERINA MARKOPOULOU, M.D.

THE NEBRASKA MEDICAL CENTER
CLARKSDN HDSPITAL - UNIVERSITY HOSPITAL
Nebraska Medical Center
Omaha NE. 68198
KOPERA. GINA M.
MRN: 00765776 SEX: F
DOB: 3Jun68
Test Date/Time: 1999-12-16:00:00
Entry/Dictating: AL-OMAISHI, JINAN
Report Name: Progress Note. Clinical
PROBLEM #2 MULTIPLE SCLEROSIS

SUBJECTIVE

Gina is a 31-year-old right-handed white female presenting for follow-up of multiple sclerosis and IV steroid burst. She was last seen on November 11, 1999. Overall she is doing quite well. She continues to have some blurring of some vision of the left eye but this is starting to resolve. She is doing well otherwise and is voicing no other concerns.

REVIEW OF SYSTEMS: There have been no significant weight changes, fever, chest pain, shortness of breath, or palpitation. She does notice that the blurring of her left eye increases with fatigue and activity. There have no problems with chewing, speaking, or swallowing. She has had no pain in her eyes. She was seen by Dr. Richard Legge on November 30 for follow-up of bilateral optic neuritis. He feels that she is going into remission. Visual acuity at that time was 20/20 on the right and 20/40 on the left and improving color vision in both eyes. She continues to have a small amount of edema in the superior pole of each optic nerve but that is resolving.

ALLERGIES: No known allergies.

Current medications: Avonex 3D meg 1M weekly, amantidine 100 mg one p.o. q. daily, Aleve p.r.n., and Triphasil 28 day one p.o. q. daily.

OBJECTIVE

Vital signs: Blood pressure is 114/64. Pulse is 76. Weight is 77.2 kg or 170 pounds.

General health: Gina is a well-developed female in no apparent acute distress. There is no change in physical evaluation from previous examination.

ASSESSMENT
Relapsing remitting multiple sclerosis. EDSS of 1 to 1.5. Flare of optic neuritis resolving.

PLAN

We will make no changes in treatment plan. We would ask that she return to clinic in approximately four months or call us in the interim if any problems arise.

We will continue Avonex 30 meg 1M weekly with monitoring lab work drawn at regular intervals.

This dictation and assessment were done in conjunction with Dr. Jinan Al-Omaishi.

MARY FILIPI, F
SIGNED 1/20/2000 1:42 PM
JINAN AL-OMAISHI. M.D.

THE NEBRASKA MEDICAL CENTER
CLARKSON HOSPITAL - UNIVERSITY HOSPITAL
Nebraska Medical Center
Omaha NE. 68198
KOPERA. GINA M.
MRN: 00765776 SEX: F
DOB: 3Jun68
Test Date/Time: 2000-05-24:00:00
Entry/Dictating: MARKOPOULOU, EKATERINI
Report Name: Progress Note. Clinical
PROBLEM #: TELEPHONE CALL

SUBJECTIVE

Gina is experiencing hematuria without symptoms of bladder infection. This has occurred suddenly. She denies any type of febrile illness with no urgency, burning or frequency. She came in and provided a urine specimen which does show results consistent with urinary tract infection. We will initiate Bactrim OS one b.i.d. x 10 days. She is to return for a repeat urinalysis in two weeks. If she continues to have hematuria, she will be referred to Urology for workup.

SIGNED 6/15/2000 6:45 PM, MARY FILIPI. F
SIGNED 6/16/2000 12:14 PM, KATERINA MARKOPOULOU. M.D.

THE NEBRASKA MEDICAL CENTER
CLARKSON HOSPITAL - UNIVERSITY HOSPITAL
Nebraska Medical Center
Omaha NE, 68198
KOPERA, GINA M,
MRN: 00765776 SEX: F
DOB: 3Jun68
Test Date/Time: 2000-09-11:00:00
Entry/Dictating: SEVERSON, MERYL
Report Name: Progress Note, Clinical

GYNECOLOGIC EXAM

ENCOUNTER VISIT: SEPTEMBER II, 2000

Gina Kopera comes in for follow-up on Ortho-Tricyclen. She

states she is happy with this. She is having regular menses, no intra menstrual spotting and has no complaints.

A prescription for Ortho-Tricyclen was written for 1 year and she is to return in June of 2001 for her annual examination.

THE NEBRASKA MEDICAL CENTER
CLARKSON HOSPITAL - UNIVERSITY HOSPITAL
Nebraska Medical Center
Omaha NE, 68198
KOPERA, GINA M.
MRN: 00765776 SEX: F
DOB: 3Jun68
Test Date/Time: 2000-06-12:00:00
Entry/Dictating: SEVERSON, MERYL
Report Name: Progress Note
GYN CLINIC VISIT
ENCOUNTER DATE: June 12, 2000

Gina Kopera comes in for annual examination today. She has multiple sclerosis and is on Avonex right now and Triphasil. She had 2 weeks of bleeding with the Triphasial and was somewhat unhappy with that.

She has no history of breast cancer in the family. She desires to continue on contraception and she stated originally that she would like to go to Depoprovera; however, after discussing this, she was on it before and stated that she went off it and it turns out that this was probably because of depression, which can be caused both by the Avonex and the Depoprovera.

EXAMINATION: Neck was supple without masses. Thyroid was negative.

Chest was symmetrical. Respirations equal bilaterally.

Breasts were normal female bilaterally. No masses, skin changes or nipple discharge. Axilla were negative bilaterally.

Abdomen was soft, flat, nontender. No masses, megaly or guarding.

Vulva was normal. Vagina was normal. Cervix appeared normal. Pap smear was obtained. Uterus was anterior, normal size, shape and consistency. Adnexa were negative for masses bilaterally.

IMPRESSION: Normal annual gynecologic examination.

PLAN: Continue oral contraceptives (after discussion, we did switch her to Orthotricyclen) and she is to return in one year or prn problems. In addition, chlamydia and gonorrhea were also obtained and she will be notified if there is any positive result. She is to return in 3 months for follow up on her new oral contraceptives.

THE NEBRASKA MEDICAL CENTER
CLARKSON HOSPITAL - UNIVERSITY HOSPITAL
Nebraska Medical Center
Omaha NE. 68198
KOPERA. GINA M.
MRN: 00765776 SEX: F
DOB: 3Jun68
Test Date/Time: 2000-07-14:00:00
Entry/Dictating: AL-OMAISHI. JINAN
Report Name: Progress Note. Clinical

PROBLEM #2 MULTIPLE SCLEROSIS

SUBJECTIVE HISTORY: Gina is a 32-year-old, right handed, white female presenting for follow-up of multiple sclerosis. At last visit Gina was not having any type of MS flares but significant family upset. She continued to take Avonex 30 mcgms 1M weekly and has done so tolerating that medication well with no side effects. Things have been working better at home, and she and her husband are now in counseling. She has lost 20 pounds in the two weeks when things were at its most stressful level and did tolerate the weight loss well, although she did have some problems with sleeping and depression.

Overall, she is feeling very well. She is feeling more rested and sleeping less. There has been no numbness or tingling noted. She occasionally will have eye sensations but denies any pain, scotoma, diplopia, or blurring of vision. She is here today for follow-up of Avonex.

There have no fevers, chest pain, palpitations, or shortness of breath. She has noted no change in bowel or bladder.

ALLERGIES:

No known allergies.

CURRENT MEDICATIONS:

Avonex 30 mcgms 1M weekly.

Ortho Tri-Cyclen one po q.d.

OBJECTIVE PHYSICAL EXAMINATION:

VITAL SIGNS:

Blood pressure is 118/74. Pulse is 68 and regular. Weight is 68.1 kg or 150.2 pounds. Temperature is 36.9.

GENERAL HEALTH:

Gina is a slender, well developed female, appearing her stated age, in no apparent acute distress.

HEENT:

Head is normocephalic without lesions or masses noted. Neck is supple with full range of motion with no thyromegaly or lymphadenopathy present. Carotids are palpable at 2/4 without bruit.

LUNGS:

Lung fields are clear with good air movement throughout.

HEART:

Heart rate is regular without murmurs or rubs.

EXTREMITIES:

Without edema.

COGNITIVE/LANGUAGE:

Language pattern is normal without dysarthria. She is alert and oriented to time. place. and person with good recent and remote recall. There are no gross cognitive deficits noted on exam.

Cranial Nerves:

I - Olfactory - Deferred.

II - Optic - Visual acuity is unchanged. Visual fields are intact.

III, IV, and VI - Oculomotor, trochlear, and abducens - Extraocular movements are intact with no nystagmus noted. Funduscopic exam is unremarkable. Pupils are equal and react well to light.

V - Trigeminal - Sensation to light touch is intact over all three branches.

VII - Facial - Facial features are symmetrical with good muscle movement throughout.

VIII - Acoustics - Gross hearing is intact.

IX, X, and XII - Glossopharyngeal, vagus, and hypoglossal - The soft palate rises to the midline. The tongue is midline without deviation or fasciculation. Gag reflex is present.

XI - Accessory nerve - Shoulder shrug is strong and equal bilaterally.

Motor/Muscle:

Muscle groups are full without atrophy, fasciculations, contractures, or rigidity. Overall body strength is excellent at 5/5. No pronator drift is noted.

Reflexes:

Reflexes are normal at 1-2/4 throughout. Hofmann and Babinski are absent.

Sensory:

There are no sensory changes noted. Pain, touch, and proprioception are intact. Romberg is absent.

Cerebellar:

Coordination testing is excellent with finger-to-nose, fine motor movement, and alternating movement. She can do heel-to-shin without difficulty.

Gait:

Gina demonstrates a narrow gait with good arm swing. She can walk on heels, toes, and tandem walk without difficulty.

ASSESSMENT:

Relapsing remitting multiple sclerosis, EDSS 1.0 to 1.5, stable on Avonex.

PLAN: We will draw monitoring lab work today of CBC and LFTs. Her last studies were normal. We will repeat these again in six months at her next follow-up visit.

This dictation and assessment were
done in conjunction with Dr. Jinan Al-Omaishi.
SIGNED 8/11/2000 11:03 AM MARY FILIPI, F
SIGNED 8/28/2000 2:06 PM JINAN AL-OMAISHI, M.D.

THE NE8RASKA MEDICAL CENTER
CLARKSON HOSPITAL - UNIVERSITY HOSPITAL
Nebraska Medical Center
Omaha NE. 68198
KOPERA. GINA M.
MRN: 00765776
Ordering ProvBREAZEALE. RICHARD
Test Date/Time: 2000-09-20:14:36
Result Status:
Dictating ProviHANKINS. JORDAN
Report Name: Tibia Fibula XR 2 Views

IMPRESSION:

1. Normal right lower leg.

FINDINGS: No bone, joint or soft tissue abnormality is seen.
No soft tissue foreign body is seen.

THE NEBRASKA MEDICAL CENTER
CLARKSON HOSPITAL - UNIVERSITY HOSPITAL
Nebraska Medical Center
Omaha NE. 6B198
KOPERA. GINA M.
MRN: 00765776 SEX: F
DOB: 3Jun68
Test Date/Time: 2001-06-04:00:00
Entry/Dictating: STANCIL, MARVIN
Report Name: Progress Note. Clinical
ENCOUNTER DATE: June 4, 2001
VITAL SIGNS: Weight is 145 pounds. Blood pressure 120/80.

SUBJECTIVE:

This 33-year-old, gravida 1, para 1-0-0-1, married white
female, last menstrual period 5/28/01, has a history of
multiple sclerosis for four years. She is doing well and is
currently on no medications for her MS. She is on oral contraceptives, Ortho TriCyclen and states that she wants to
stop this method. She at this point has no desire for additional children but she is not adamant about that. After

discussion of various birth control options, she elects to be off all hormonal contraception and wants to proceed with IUD insertion. Her last menstrual period was six days and it was a normal flow. She has no contraindications to IUD. She is monogamous, has no past history of STD's PID and after discussion of this method elects to proceed with this insertion today.

OBJECTIVE:

Breasts are soft, nontender. no mass. She does have bilateral saline implants. The abdomen is soft and nontender without mass. She has healed incision from two previous cesarean sections. Extremities are unremarkable. Pelvic examination revealed normal external genitalia, vagina and cervix. Cultures for GC and chlamydia were obtained. The uterus is anteverted, parous, nontender. The adnexa is clear bilaterally. After betadine prep the uterine cavity was sounded to 7 cm. A Paragar IUD was inserted without difficulty and the IUD string was cut approximately 1.5 cm from the cervix. The patient tolerated this insertion well.

ASSESSMENT:

1. Normal annual examination.

2. IUD insertion.

PLAN: She is to return to clinic in 1-2 months for IUD follow up. She will stop oral contraceptives effective immediately.

Dictated by Marvin Stancil. MD

THE NEBRASKA MEDICAL CENTER
CLARKSON HOSPITAL - UNIVERSITY HOSPITAL
Nebraska Medical Center
Omaha NE. 68198
KOPERA. GINA M.
MRN: 00765776 SEX: F
DOB: 3Jun68
Test Date/Time: 2001-07-02:00:00

Entry/Dictating: STANCIL, MARVIN
Report Name: Progress Note. Clinical
ENOUNTER DATE: July 2, 2001
VITAL SIGNS: Weight was 139 pounds. Blood pressure 120/80.

SUBJECTIVE:

This 33-year-old gravida 1, para 1, white female, child is five years old, had an IUD placed one month ago. She had just recently stopped oral contraceptives. During this past month she states that she has had cramping and pain with intercourse as well as her partner being able to feel the IUD string and she wants the IUD out. Options of management were discussed with her including trimming the IUD string and also evaluation for endometritis and antibiotic therapy. The patient states that she has definitely decided she want IUD out and will return to oral contraceptives pending her partner having a vasectomy. She has no contraindication to oral contraceptives. She does smoke 10 cigarettes per day.

OBJECTIVE:

An IUD string was visible and the IUD was removed. Pelvic examination revealed no cervical motion tenderness. The uterus is anteverted and somewhat tender to palpation. The adnexa is clear.

ASSESSENT:

1. Elects to have IUD removed.

2. Possible endometritis.

PLAN: The patient is given Doxycycline 100 mg po bid for seven days. She has no allergies. Motrin 800 mg q 6-8 hours PRN pain, #30 tablets. Ortho TriCyclen with refills for one year. She is told to return to clinic PRN.

Dictated by Marvin Stancil. MD
Cc: Dr. Harrison
Gail Hille. Nurse Practitioner

THE NEBRASKA MEDICAL CENTER
CLARKSON HOSPITAL - UNIVERSITY HOSPITAL
Nebraska Medical Center
Omaha NE, 68198
KOPERA, GINA M.
SEX: F
DOB: 3Jun68
Test Date/Time: 2001-08-08:00:00
Report Name: Progress Note, Clinical
Entry/Dictating: FILIPI, MARY
NEUROLOGY CLINIC - PROGRESS NOTE
ENCOUNTER DATE: July 27, 2001
COLLABORATING PHYSICIAN: Ekaterini Markopoulou, MD

DIAGNOSIS:

Multiple sclerosis.

SUBJECTIVE:

Gina is a 33-year-old right-handed white female presenting for followup with multiple sclerosis with clinical progression. She was last seen July 14, 2000. Gina had been
on Avonex for treatment of the disease but stopped that in
November 2000 due to cost and her desire to be off of all
medications. She felt she has been symptom-free and saw
no need to proceed with medication. She had made some
dietary changes, eliminating wheat and gluten from her
diet, and had felt much better. She had also lost significant
weight. She began having eye problems in June, developing
blindness in the left eye. Two weeks ago, the left fingers became uncoordinated and made her work as a hair dresser
more difficult. She has seen improvement since that time.
She also began having problems with the right hand after
this. She was dropping items and developing a shakiness.
Gina had also had some extreme discomfort in the stomach
and abdomen which is gone now, She has recently had her
eyes checked by Dr. Stephanie Meyer. Gina connects a lot of

her problems to the removal of an IUD. She became infected shortly after the IUD removal and has been on antibiotics.

There have been no fevers, chest pain, or palpitations. She has noted no change in bowel or bladder habits. She continues to be sexually active with no perineal sensation changes. There had been significant amount of marital upset and that seems to have leveled off. Her and her husband are cohabiting again and she feels this is working well.

Allergies: No known allergies.

Current medications: None.

OBJECTIVE:

Vital signs: Blood pressure 110/60, pulse 64 and regular, weight is 61.6 kg.

Gina is a slender well-developed female appearing her stated age in no apparent acute distress. Head is normocephalic without lesions or masses noted. Neck is supple with full range of motion with no thyromegaly or lymphadenopathy present. Carotids are palpable at 2/4 without bruits. Lung fields are clear with good air movement throughout. Heart rate is regular without murmur or rub. Extremities are without edema.

Cognitive/Language: Language pattern is normal without dysarthria. She is alert and oriented to time, place, and person with good recent and remote recall. There are no gross cognitive deficits noted on exam.

Cranial Nerves:

I: Olfactory - deferred.

II: Optic - visual acuity is 20/25 bilaterally with contacts. Visual fields are intact.

III, IV, VI: Oculomotor, trochlear, abducens - extraocular

movements are intact with no nystagmus noted. A Marcus Gunn is present on the left. There is a paleness to the disc and some atrophy by funduscopic exam.

V: Trigeminal - there is decreased sensation in the left lower branch. This was present approximately one month ago.

VII: Facial - facial features are symmetrical with good muscle movement throughout.

VIII: Acoustic - gross hearing is intact.

IX, X, XII: Glossopharyngeal, vagus, hypoglossal - the soft palate rises to the midline. there is a right deviation of the tongue. Gag reflex is present.

XI: Accessory nerve - shoulder shrug is strong and equal bilaterally.

Motor/Muscle: Muscle groups are full without atrophy, fasciculations, contractures, or rigidity. Upper body strength is excellent at 5/5. Hip flexors are 4+/5 on the right, 5/5 on the left, with extensor, dorsi, and plantar flexion at 5/5 bilaterally.

Reflexes: Upper body reflexes are normal at 1/4 to 2/4. Patellar reflexes are 4/4 bilaterally with ankle jerk at a 1/4 to 2/4 bilaterally. Hoffman and Babinski are absent.

Sensory: There is decreased vibration sense over all, left greater than right; and no proprioception on the left hand. She also identifies a decreased sensation to pinprick on the left hand with a gross sensory level. She also identifies a T3-4 truncal sensory level: this is a change since her previous exam. Romberg is absent.

Cerebellar: There is a overshoot and correct with finger-to-nose on the left. She is able to do fine motor movement and alternating movement without difficulty. Heel-to-shin is normal without signs of ataxia.

Gait: Gina demonstrates a narrow gait with good arm swing. She can walk on heels, toes, and tandem walk.

ASSESSMENT:

1. Relapsing, remitting multiple sclerosis with clinical progression.

2. Uterine infection following IUD (intrauterine device) removal.

PLAN:

We would like to obtain an MRI of the brain, cervical, and thoracic spine due to the sensory levels noted. She is to follow up with us after testing is complete for discussion of further treatment plan. We would highly recommend that she return to the use of one of the modulating agents but this will be assessed after MRI is done.

This dictation and assessment were done
in conjunction with Dr. Ekaterini Markopoulou.
Dictated by Mary F. Filipi. ARNP/sjf
This report was reprinted from the electronic Medical Record

APPENDIX C

LiveJuice Recipes

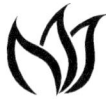

When you begin juicing, for a fast or even while eating it helps to see some sample recipes to giving you ideas of where to start. After you have been juicing for a while, you will get more creative and come up with your very own recipes using the vegetables and fruits that you like.

The juice from the food you have eaten is the main source of the nutrition. As your body is digesting food you have eaten, the digestive juices begin extraction of juice from the food. The body also works to separate the bulk from the juice. This is the power of live juice fasting, there is no extra work for your body to do.

The remaining bulk of food then goes out as waste, while the juice is utilized by the body for nutrition. If you swallow juice without chewing it first, it will decrease the effectiveness of the live juice you are drinking. Treat live juice as solid food. Chew the live juice as this starts your digestion process. Chewing action mixes the juice with your saliva. This prepares it for your digestive system allowing the fresh live juice to enter your bloodstream with a blast of nutrition.

It takes 60% of your energy and sometimes hours to digest food. When you juice the body no longer needs to break down the food that you ate. The result from the juice is immediately released into the bloodstream. When you have a weak-ened digestive system, this will certainly give it the break that it deserves.

Simply remember, any strong medicine does not taste good. Juicing is not about pleasing your taste buds.

JuicePower and Mucous-Free Juice Recipes

These are more recipes that are much tastier. A great way to start out to get the idea of what juicing is all about. If you can always get organic, it more nutritious plus tastes more flavorful. If you cannot purchase organic or grow on your own, anything is better than nothing at all.

To clean your vegetables use 2 tablespoons of apple cider vinegar in a sink or bowl full of cold water, let it sit for 5 minutes, then rinse off with cold water. This assists getting any residue off your produce.

You can use these combinations, as a foundation and keep building from here:

5 carrots
1 apple (I throw in the whole apple, stem and all. Some say you should not juice the seeds. I do and I am not dead yet!)

-----

5 carrots
1 apple
ginger root (slice a piece the size of your thumbnail, you will find that this gets spicy the more you add)

-----

1 beet
1 apple
1 carrot
¼ of fennel

¼ to ½ lemon
2 to 4 apples
    Don't forget to juice the lemon peel for extra nutrition.

½ zucchini
4 carrots

½ apple

-----

5 or 6 carrots

handful of spinach

1 kale leaf

½ red or green pepper

2 Brussels sprouts

½ to 1 apple

-----

1 parsnip

¼ turnip

A small handful of turnip greens

2 to 4 celery stalks

2 to 4 apples

¼ to ½ grapefruit

1 to 2 apples

½ pineapple +rind

    The rind contains a lot of beneficial nutrition including the digestive enzyme known as "bromelain". And it taste great!

-----

watermelon + rind

    Great diuretic, you also want the watermelon with seeds as the seeds have a plenty of nutritional value.

PowerHouse Juice Recipes

With the PowerHouse fast, your main aim is to eliminate sugar; it does not matter what form it is in, sugar is sugar. Cucumber is the base for these green juice recipes. For a green vegetable it is sweeter than other green vegetables without all the carbs, and more palatable.

If you can, always buy organic. It is more nutritious plus is more flavorful. If you cannot purchase organic or grow on your own, anything is better than nothing at all.

To clean your vegetables use 2 tablespoons of apple cider vinegar in a sink or bowl full of cold water. Let it sit for 5 minutes, then rinse off with cold water. This assists getting residue off your produce.

> Helpful Trick: Improve your live juice, if bitter, by adding CayennePower. It will make the juice palatable.

You can use these combinations, as a foundation and keep building from here:

1 Cucumber

-----

1 Cucumber
¼ of Lemon squeezed or juiced

> Treat lemon as a spice. As it does have approximately 21 grams of Carbohydrate in a whole lemon. I leave the skin on when I put it through the juicer and some don't. If peeling the skin off, leave some of the white membrane on the fruit. The membrane of the lemon contains the bioflavonoid. Bioflavonoid helps the bodies absorb and use Vitamin C.

-----

1 cucumber
fennel (cut a ¼ of the bulb, I put the whole stalk in too)

-----

1 cucumber
1 stalk of celery
green onion (put the whole thing in)

-----

1 cucumber
garlic (1 or more cloves)
4 drops of CayennePower

-----

1 cucumber
garlic (1 or more cloves)
several drops of CayennePower

-----

fennel (cut a ¼ of the bulb, I put the whole stalk in too)
1 cucumber
ginger root (cut a piece the size of your thumbnail)
some spinach (start with several pieces, then add more as you get use to it)
1 green onion (put the whole thing in)

-----

1 cucumber
¼ of a cabbage
several drops of CayennePower

-----

1 cucumber
cilantro (several sprigs)
green onion (put the whole thing in)

-----

6 stalks of celery
(Helped me overcome insomnia)

Works Cited

Michio Kushi, and Stephen Blauer. The Macrobiotic Way The Complete Macrobiotic Diet & Exercise Book. New York: Avery, 1984.

Balch, James F. Prescription for Nutritional Healing. 2nd ed. Garden City Park, N.Y: Avery Pub. Group, 1997.

Batmanghelidj, Fereydoon. Your Body's Many Cries for Water You Are Not Sick, You Are Thirsty. Deerfield Beach: Global Health Solutions, 1997.

Beckett, Ann. "First Do No Harm." First Do No Harm. 16 Feb. 1997.

Biser, Sam. Curing with Cayenne. Van Nuys: Save Your Life Videos, Inc., 2000.

Biser, Sam. "Sam Biser." Sam Biser. <http://www.sambiser.com/>.

Christopher, John R. Herbal Home Health Care. Springville, Utah: Christopher Publications, 1976.

Christopher, John R. School of Natural Healing. Minneapolis: Christopher Publications (UT), 1996.

Clark, Hulda Regehr. Cure for all diseases with many case histories of diabetes, high blood pressure, seizures, chronic fatigue syndrome, migraines, Alzheimer's, Parkinson's, multiple sclerosis, and others showing that all of these can be simply investigated and cured. San Diego, CA: New Century P, 1995.

Crook, William G. Yeast connection a medical breakthrough. New York: Vintage Books, 1986.

D'Adamo, Peter J. Eat Right 4 Your Type The Individualized Diet Solution to Staying Healthy, Living Longer & Achieving Your Ideal Weight. New York: Putnam Adult, 1996.

"Dietary Goals for the United States (1977) and Diet, Nutrition and Cancer (1982)."

"Dr. Christopher." http://www.herballegacy.com/. School of Natural Healing. <http://www.herballegacy.com/>.

Dr. Hulda Carke. <http://www.drclark.net/>.

Dr. Lorraine Day. <http://www.drday.com/>.

Dyer, Wayne W. The Wayne Dyer CD Collection [ABRIDGED]. New York: Hay House, 2002.

Fallon, Sally. Nourishing traditions the cookbook that challenges politically correct nutrition and the diet dictocrats. Washington, DC: NewTrends Pub., 1999.

"Herbs and Supplies." Mountain Rose Herbs. <http://www.mountainroseherbs. com/>.

"Herbs and Supplies." Starwest-Botanicals. <http://www.starwest-botanicals. com/>.

"Herbs." Blessed Herbs. <http://www.blessedherbs.com/bh/?s_hsplt=1>.

"Herbs." Pacific Botanicals. <http://www.pacificbotanicals.com/>.

Moskowitz, Isa Chandra, and Terry Hope Romero. Veganomicon The Ultimate Vegan Cookbook. Boston: Marlowe & Company, 2007.

Myers, Joyce. Battlefield of the Mind. Cal: Warner Faith, 1995.

"Raw Milk." Weston A. Price. Weston A. Price Foundation. <http://www. westonaprice.org/>.

Schulze, Dr. Richard. "Dr. Schulzes Web Page." Dr. Schulze's. American Botanical Pharmacy. <https://web0.herbdoc.com/index.php?&c=1>.

Schulze, Dr. Richard. Healing Naturally. Marina del Ray: Natural Healing publish-cations, 2006.

"Supplies." Supplies. <http://www.essentialsupplies.com/~smartcart/index.cgi>.

ABOUT THE AUTHOR

Gina Kopera is a Master Herbalist, Midwest-based researcher, author, consultant, and coach in the field of Alternative Health. She is also the president of Gina's Corner devoted to informing MS patients and others about effective alternative therapies and helping them take advantage of those therapies.

Gina's interest in alternative health began when she was a teenager. Serious back problems meant she saw numerous doctors, tried 19 prescription drugs, and missed a fair amount of school. It seemed the only option left was surgery. Her father was against major back surgery and instead took her to a nutritionist. What followed was a regime of diet and exercise. In three months the pain was gone with no recurrence. This proved to be just the first time traditional western medicine could not help Gina with major medical conditions.

As an adult she suffered years of painful and debilitating symptoms from remitting and relapsing MS, eventually turning back to natural alternatives to restore her health. Gina has used the natural remedies in this book to cure herself of MS symptoms and her son of epilepsy symptoms.

Her passion is teaching others effective natural alternatives to help others empower themselves and take control of their own lives; bringing health and happiness back again.

Gina Kopera is living in Council Bluffs, Iowa with her family.

www.ingramcontent.com/pod-product-compliance
Lightning Source LLC
Chambersburg PA
CBHW070809270326
41927CB00010B/2366